GII00381246

VIRAL
SELF
DEFENCE

AND THE SCIENCE BEHIND IT

VIRAL SELF DEFENCE

AND THE SCIENCE BEHIND IT

SARA DAVENPORT

REBOOT
PRESS

To all the frontline health workers and social carers battling so heroically on our behalf in these unprecedented times

With heartfelt thanks.

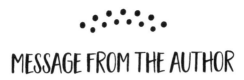

MESSAGE FROM THE AUTHOR

This is my own personal 'clapping for the carers' effort, to raise funds for doctors, nurses and hospital staff in need in these difficult times, and for all the social carers working so courageously in nursing homes around the country, keeping the sick and the elderly safe.

100% of the proceeds of sales from the book will be donated to the Cavell Trust (Reg charity no 1160148). Your money will go to the frontline health professionals for financial emergencies and your generosity in contributing towards this fund is hugely appreciated.

In 'Viral Self Defence' I have put together as much science backed information as I could find to create what I hope will be a useful reference manual for us all, now and in the future.

Keeping your immune system strong is the key to both avoiding, and recovering faster, from viral infection. The evidence for anti-viral natural health remedies is extensive and they have been successfully used throughout the centuries in countries across the globe. We need all the help we can get at present, and nature offers wide-ranging solutions that work successfully, and without side-effects, alongside conventional medicine.

Thank you so much for buying the book. Together, I hope we can all make a difference and support the enormous generosity of the carers, protecting the rest of us at great personal risk.

Let's stay safe.

Sara x

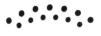

CONTENTS

INTRODUCTION 1

CHAPTER ONE: ALL ABOUT VIRUSES 3
    What is a virus? 3
    The difference between bacteria and viruses 4
    How viruses attack 5
    How viruses spread 6
    What is viral load? 8

CHAPTER TWO: HOW TO AVOID A VIRUS 9
    Develop new habits 9
    Protective masks..14
    Try not to panic 15
    Instant access to a doctor..15

CHAPTER THREE: YOUR IN-BUILT ANTI-VIRAL PROTECTION 17
    It's all about your Immune System................................17
    Understanding the difference between your
    'immune system' and 'immunity'....................................18
    The white blood cells..19
    The problem with viruses 21

CHAPTER FOUR: IMMUNE SYSTEM ACTION PLAN 22
    The Three Keys:
    1: Establish the strength of your immune System..23
    2: Unload what weakens your immune system.......25
    3: Boost Your Immune System..30

CHAPTER FIVE: SLEEP ACTION PLAN 45

How long should you sleep? 45

Keep a Sleep Diary...46

Pre-bed sleep habits 48

Quick fix sleep techniques 49

CHAPTER SIX: EXERCISE ACTION PLAN.................................. 52

Why you need to exercise.................................... 52

How to get your muscles moving 53

High intensity interval training 54

Online apps..56

CHAPTER SEVEN: ANTI-VIRAL NUTRITIONAL SUPPLEMENTS 58

What to take and why? 58

My Daily Dose of Anti-viral Supplements................ 62

IV Therapy 63

CHAPTER EIGHT: HARNESS THE POWER OF PLANTS..............................66

Anti-viral essential oils 67

Plants: The Heavy Hitters.................................... 70

CHAPTER NINE: AIR, OZONE AND HEAT 76

Clean up your Air... 76

Oxygen Healing 77

Oxidation 80

Ozone 80

Heat.. 82

CHAPTER TEN: MAKE YOUR OWN ANTI-VIRAL HOME SOLUTIONS..........87

Anti-viral surface cleaner..87

Anti-viral hand sanitiser..89

Anti-viral room spray..90

Anit-viral fruit and vegetable cleaner..........................92

CHAPTER ELEVEN: EMOTIONS AND IMMUNITY......................................93

Anti-viral Emotional Defence..94

Design a Day to Day Timetable......................................95

Get technology savvy..97

Isolation..98

Strategies for working from home..............................99

CHAPTER TWELVE: STRESS RELIEF: UNLOAD YOUR BURDEN.................101

Establish your current stress levels............................102

Identify Your Stresses – Past and Present...............103

How to reduce stress...108

CHAPTER THIRTEEN: CORONAVIRUS – A GLOBAL PANDEMIC................119

COVID-19 Facts And Figures...119

The R0 number..120

Animal contagion...121

COVID-19 Symptoms...122

Potential medical solutions..124

Complementary therapies for Coronavirus
symptoms relief..126

ENDNOTES..142

INDEX..151

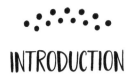

INTRODUCTION

Modern medicine has few pharmaceutical solutions that offer an effective defence against existing viral infections – whether it is stopping the annual influenza virus in its tracks, alleviating shingles, herpes or HPV, or dealing with more serious outbreaks such as SARS, H5N1 bird flu or MERS. Attempting to limit the spread of the current Covid-19 pandemic that has affected every country around the globe is currently stretching our resources to the limit.

The battle between mankind and the virus has been waged over centuries. The likelihood is that in the years to come ever more previously unknown infectious viruses will emerge to infect us globally and with stretches of time needed to develop vaccines against them, we all need an effective fallback to bridge the gap.

Boosting the immune system is key to fending off infection and reducing the severity of any symptoms should infection take hold. This book is an attempt to offer evidence-based support to bolster the medical options available by gathering together natural remedies proven over time to damage and destroy viruses and strengthen the immune system[1]. Complementary and conventional medicine, working together, hand in hand, can make each of us more resilient.

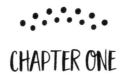

CHAPTER ONE

ALL ABOUT VIRUSES

What is a virus?

Viruses are unlike the majority of other life forms on this planet. They do not have cells, they can't reproduce themselves, and they don't produce their own energy. All of these are fundamental requirements for our definition of life, so precisely what they are remains a conundrum. Do they even qualify as 'alive'?

Viruses are simple structures, made up of a set of genes enclosed in a protective protein shell called a capsid, and some have an additional layer around them, called an envelope. Since they don't have cells that can reproduce to multiply, they can only replicate themselves inside the living cells of other organisms, taking over much in the same way that a cuckoo occupies another songbirds nest.

Whatever their state of being (or not being), viruses have been present alongside us for millenia, and although some have proved beneficial to human beings, the majority bring infection, disease and frequently death in their wake. Throughout history, sometimes with intervals of hundreds of years, new viruses have emerged, and old ones have mutated, that have caused devastation to vast swathes of the population[1]. The Spanish Flu pandemic of 1918-19 was triggered by a virus, killing between 20 and 40 million people across the world. Similarly, the HIV/AIDS virus killed approximately 1.5m people in a period of 12 months in 2013. SARS, H1N1 (Swine Flu) and MERS are more recent examples of what happens when a virus infects a population that has no immunity against it. Less virulently, the influenza virus affects large swathes of the population each winter, mutating slightly each season to successfully avoid destruction by the immunisation vaccines produced to shield against it in laboratories across the globe.

There are currently more than 400 different viruses that can cause infections, including the common cold, herpes, hepatitis and HIV.

The difference between bacteria and viruses

Bacteria, unlike viruses, are definitely 'alive'. They are single-celled organisms with an exterior membrane encapsulating a liquid interior. They can reproduce on their own and survive in almost any circumstance – hot or cold, and however inhospitable – anywhere in the world and there are thought to be more than 5 million trillion trillion, if you can get your head around that number, of them in existence.[2] Less than 1% of bacteria are harmful for human beings, although the Plague or Black Death of the 14th century was bacterial in origin.

Infections are caused either by bacteria or by viruses. Bacterial infections, for example, include strep throat, urinary tract infections and tuberculosis. Viral infections include the common cold, chickenpox or AIDS, and some illnesses, such as diarrhoea, meningitis or pneumonia can be triggered by either. Whereas bacterial infections are usually limited to a single area of the body, viral infections affect the whole body. One crucial difference is that whilst bacteria can be treated effectively with anti-biotics, which target certain parts of the bacteria in the hopes of killing them, if you are under viral attack there's nothing any GP can do for you except tell you to go home, rest and wait for the symptoms to pass. Anti-viral medicines can do little except attempt to prevent the viruses multiplying further.[3]

How viruses attack

Viruses attach themselves to the outer membrane of a cell and then invade it if your immune system is weak and your body has no defences at the ready to repel them. Those of us who are older, frail or with pre-existing serious health conditions are more vulnerable to viral illness than those with stronger immune systems. Because viruses are continually changing and adapting it is hard to develop drugs and vaccines against them.

There are anti-viral drugs, which interfere with the virus' reproduction cycles, stopping them from multiplying, but often not killing them off. Ultraviolet light has been shown to kill germs, and equally, some die when frozen, though others are just slowed by the process, and come back to life when thawed. Viruses are hard to destroy, and your own body is the most experienced 'viral eradicator' – if, and only if, you give it the tools to keep your immune system in prime working order.

If your immune system is strong it should be able to reduce symptoms or prevent infection altogether. *Keeping your immunity high is crucial in any effort to recover rapidly from an attack.*

How viruses spread

Viruses spread rapidly from person to person in a variety of ways. They can travel through the air, invisibly, via droplets and small particles from sneezing or coughing. Some move via contaminated foods, dirty hands or polluted water. Others are carried by insects and can be transferred by bites; others travel in bodily fluids. You can catch them from people nearby you in a crowded place, in a restaurant or bar, at a football match or concert – or from anyone coughing close to you on the buses or the tube or from someone spitting in the street. Or simply by walking down a busy road. You can pick them up from touching an infected surface – a cash machine in the bank, a door handle, light switch or from the money in your wallet that's been passed from hand to hand.

If you are infected by a virus, expect to fall 'under the weather' rapidly. Viruses replicate by hijacking the healthy cells in your body and using them to multiply and spread. And as rapidly as modern medicine comes up with pharmaceutical products to neutralise their efforts, currently those viruses remain one step ahead and continue to mutate faster.

On top of fending off viral infection, your defence system has to deal daily with your less than perfect cells - the 'senescent' cells – the ageing, abnormal or cancerous cells that can turn rogue and mutate, harming rather than helping you. The key players in your immune system are your white blood cells – and the most important of these are the Natural Killer cells (NK cells), the T-cells and the B-cells. In normal circumstances they work efficiently together as a team, destroying unidentifiable invaders and cleaning up older malfunctioning cells.

When your body gets overwhelmed by stress, however, and remains in that state over a long period of time, these cells stop functioning efficiently and their numbers go down, allowing inflammation, infection and ultimately, more serious health issues to overwhelm your system. The lower your NK cell activity the higher your risk of falling prey to a viral infection.

It's a modern day Catch-22: impossible not to be stressed both mentally and physically by the onset of viral infection, and yet so much harder to recover unless you can reduce both those types of stress.

What is viral load?

In a nutshell it means keeping your exposure to any virus as minimal as possible so that your immune system can systematically deal with it and get rid of it from your body. The prime minister, whilst discussing the COVID-19 pandemic, talks about 'flattening the curve', protecting the NHS from collapse by controlling the trajectory of the infection spread, and viral load is your own personal version of the concept.

One or two microbes picked up from the air may be manageable, but sit next to an infected person on the bus, cram yourself into a crowded tube or train, go to a concert or a football match, and you may well return home with literally billions of the viruses having infected you, with your immune system more than likely to collapse under the onslaught.

That's why keeping the concept of 'viral load' at the forefront of your mind can be literally life-saving. And anything you can do to keep it low will help you get through more successfully, your immune system remaining stronger and more resilient and protecting you more efficiently.

CHAPTER TWO

ACTION PLAN: HOW TO AVOID A VIRUS

C hanging your day to day behaviour is the top recommended anti-viral defence strategy. Taking a few simple steps has been shown to reduce infection rates and slow the spread of contagion.

Develop new habits

Track your temperature - 'Normal' temperatures can vary from person to person. Invest in a thermometer and establish your own personal baseline. Keep a daily watch out for any changes. The average normal body temperature is 37°C (98.6°F) but there is a wider range also considered 'healthy' – fluctuating from 36.1°C (97°F) to 37.2°C (99°F). A temperature over 38°C (100.4°F) may indicate you have a fever caused by illness or infection.

Wash your hands frequently and stop touching your face - We apparently touch our faces with our hands an average of 23 times an hour, transferring any bacteria or virus from the environment to our mouths, eyes, nose and ears in the process.[1]

Touch a virus laden-kitchen surface, count a wad of notes or pick through the coins of your wallet or purse and you are unlikely to escape contamination. Credit card machines, mobile phones, door handles and simply shaking hands can transfer literally billions of unknown viruses from one person to another. And viruses can survive for several hours and replicate themselves during that period, multiplying exponentially.[2] The best thing to do is keep washing your hands throughout the day, with soap and water, for at least 20 seconds each time, and keep a pack of anti-bacterial wipes close by.

Take additional care if you are coughing or sneezing - Carry a handkerchief or tissue with you at all times, and cough or sneeze into that rather than into your bare hands. It's not just about how other people's germs could affect you, but also how you could pass contagion on to others around you. Become more conscious of your own habits and actions and take greater care around your neighbours.

Clean your TV remotes, door handles and taps regularly - You can't pick up an infection simply by touching a contaminated surface, only if you touch it and then go on to rub your eyes or touch your mouth or nose. Think light switches, keyboards, hairdryers and kitchen gadgets.

Bin your old multi-use cleaning cloths that can provide an environment for viruses to breed in or soak them in diluted bleach after each use. Keep your kitchen surfaces clean and again, use bleach, which destroys viruses fast, to disinfect your toilet seats and flush handles. Dilute the bleach to one-part bleach: ten-parts water. Dettol is also effective. Close the toilet seat before you flush to stop the virus spraying around the room – and for the same reason, try not to use the hot-air-drying machines in public bathrooms but paper towels instead. A Mayo clinic research review concluded that 'from a hygiene viewpoint, paper towels are superior to electric air dryers'.[3]

Tests on these machines talk of 'spreading faecal matter'. Viral transmission is more likely to occur from wet skin than from dry skin, so make sure your hands are properly dried.

Limit your TV and newspaper time - Worrying about an invisible virus that none of us know very much about is definitely stressful, and as panic fills the pages of the newspapers and the television screens, it is likely to cumulatively raise blood pressure, depress our immune systems and make us more susceptible to infection. Try to limit the feelings of panic and restrict your 'bad news' exposure to a short period – and once a day rather than repeatedly.

Avoid large groups of people - Keep your contact with others to a minimum. Most viruses are contagious, some much more than others and for longer than others. Symptoms do not emerge for 5 days initially, leaving people highly infectious during that period. Stay away from packed sporting events, concerts, theatres and cinemas and avoid crowded buses and trains where you can.

Be careful in close contact meetings - Shaking hands or kissing on the cheek is out. Try a wave, nod or smile instead. Don't share drinking cups, water bottles or knives and forks. Avoid having visitors to your home. When you have to go out, to the supermarket or the pharmacy, Government advice is to try to keep a 2m distance from other people.

Swap to contactless money - Think how many people must have touched those bank notes before you, so if you are still using coins or cash, wash your hands more frequently and use your credit card contactlessly whenever possible. Use an antibacterial wipe to wipe it down regularly after use.

Clean your mobile phone and ipads daily - Invest in a pack of spectacle and lens wipes for smear free cleaning. Make sure you have turned them off, then dampen a cloth with washing up liquid and water, squeezing it out thoroughly first. Use an alcohol wipe on the surface to quickly dry it. And don't forget their cases...

Wash all fruits and vegetables - As with your hands, wash fruit and vegetables with soap and water thoroughly before you eat them because soap seems to be able to penetrate the membrane of the virus and kill it. Combine vinegar and bicarbonate of soda with water to wash all cans and bottles – the liquid will fizz up and penetrates into the nooks and crannies. See p92.

Consider postponing travel plans - Think carefully before getting on a plane or taking a cruise. Apart from being forced into close proximity with people who may have come from virus infected areas, the real danger here is in the recycled air that must contain billions, if not trillions, of invisible viruses and bacteria.

> **Top Tip:** If you do need to travel, invest in a small and inexpensive ionic air filtration system that you can hang around your neck and will allow you to breathe pure air into your lungs. The AirTamer Personal Air Purifier (airtamer.com) cleans the air directly around you by removing viruses, bacteria and pollen.

And last but certainly not least – think of ways to help your neighbours and elderly relatives - Older people are the most vulnerable to viral contagion, and many are confined to their homes with little or no social interaction or help. Call them regularly for a chat, or drop off shopping they may struggle to get out for. Collect their prescriptions or their pension for them if they cannot.

Thinking about wearing a protective mask?

The current advice is - don't waste your money. The white ones are ineffective because they simply don't filter small enough particles. They are not designed to block viral particles and don't lie flush to your face. They will, however, protect you from any droplets from a virally infected person.

If you are going to invest, spend a bit more and make sure you check your chosen mask's anti-haze number. The higher it is, the more it's going to protect you. If it says N95 on it, it's going to filter out 95% of airborne particulates.

Top Tip: The R-pur is a French-made mask that removes 99.98% of even the finest of particulates. (R-pur.com).

A newly developed 'snood' mask from virustaticshield.com[4], is about to go into production, made from fabric with an anti-viral coating that blocks airborne droplets and kills any microbes carried in them. Researchers at Imperial College, London tested the snoods, pushing air containing viruses through the material. Results showed that 96% of the viruses were destroyed.

Non-thermal plasma masks which are currently still in development look like being an effective way of controlling viral infection. New research shows that 99.9% of harmful viruses are de-activated by this cold plasma technology which enters bacteria, viruses and fungi and destroys the free DNA of the microbes inside the cells, killing them.[5]

> **Top Tip:** Be careful whilst filling up at the petrol station. Carry anti-bacterial wipes to disinfect the petrol pump; wear gloves, or use paper towels and bin them straight away.

Try not to panic

Panic is contagious. Internet rumours and media frenzy can trigger fear, confusion and intense anxiety in a whole population far faster than any virus can spread. Colder months are always a time of coughs, colds and viruses and because you are sneezing and spluttering and feeling generally terrible, does not necessarily mean you may have come in contact with the coronavirus.

Instant access to a doctor

Worried about your symptoms and can't get through to your normal GP practise? Sign up for one of the on-line surgeries and get access to a doctor from the comfort of your own home. Choosing an on-line appointment removes the need to sit for hours in a waiting room crowded with sick people, with the uneasy thought that you may come out having caught something you didn't go in with and end up sicker than when you started. Many doctors surgeries in the UK don't take calls or emails on a weekend either – several of these operate 24/7. Push Doctor (pushdoctor. co.uk), employs 100 or more ex NHS doctors and each 10 minute appointment costs £20 plus a £3 a month ongoing fee. The GP service (thegpservice.co.uk), i-gp (i-gp.uk) and Babylon Health (babylonhealth.com) offer similar services.

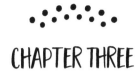

CHAPTER THREE

YOUR IN-BUILT ANTI-VIRAL PROTECTION

It's all about your Immune System

Your ability to stay well directly correlates to the strength of your immune system, and whether it has the capacity to fend off a viral invasion, from the mildest common cold or winter flu, through to a bout of shingles, an attack of norovirus or a more serious epidemic such as the coronavirus breakouts of SARS, MERS and now COVID-19.

Over-use of antibiotics has led to an increase in anti-biotic resistant bacteria, and viruses do not respond to these drugs at all. Conventional medicines solution for viral infection is to develop vaccines, but these take time to get to the mass market and often have side effects. Anti-viral drugs may reduce symptoms but generally need to be taken right at the beginning of any illness, and also have contra-indications. In the meantime, prevention by boosting your immune system is a hopeful way forward.

Your immune system is made up of billions of white blood cells and also includes the bone marrow, antibodies and your thymus gland. It is in charge of attacking and destroying the millions of microbes (bacteria, viruses, parasites and fungi) that flood your body each and every day. Your overall health relies on the success of the constant battle between your immune system - your personal invisible defence system - and these external attackers. It's a never-ending battle between warring factions and the stronger your army the greater your chance of a long and healthy life.

Your immune system is boosted when you remove or reduce what is weakening it, and then add in what makes it strong. It's that simple.

Understanding the difference between your 'immune system' and 'immunity'

Immune system

The immune system is your own inbuilt defence against invading microbes – bacteria, viruses, fungi and parasites. Different organs, cells and chemicals all work together, linked by large numbers of white blood cells, to make up an army set up specifically to prevent you getting sick. When it is functioning optimally your immune system can tell the difference between what belongs inside your body naturally, and what is attacking it from outside. It remembers every germ that it has ever defeated and creates 'antibodies' to ensure that it has the ability to recognise them should they return and immediately destroy them fast.

It is made up of:

- *The lymphatic system* – which contains lymph nodes, which trap and contain any foreign pathogens; lymphocytes - the white blood cells that track down any external attacks or breaches in its defences; and the lymph fluid that carries armies of virus fighting white blood cells around your body.

- *The spleen* – this is the factory that makes the antibodies that fight the microbes and the lymphocytes that make up your anti-viral army. It also disposes of any dead invading germs.

- *The complement system* - made up of types of proteins that work alongside antibodies.

- *The thymus* – which produces the T-lymphocyte white blood cells.

- *The bone marrow* - the spongy tissue inside your bones which produces additional white blood cells for fighting off infection.

The white blood cells

Your white blood cells, your leukocytes, are the key to your defence against viral invasion. They are your foot soldiers, constantly on patrol. When they track down foreign pathogens they multiply immediately and send out instructions to other types of cells to do the same. They divide into two main camps – the phagocytes which surround and defeat any attackers, effectively eating and then removing them, and the lymphocytes which log the invaders and prevent any future re-attack. Lymphocytes are divided into the B-cells (which produce antibodies), the T-cells, which destroy any cells that have been damaged by the viral attack and NK cells (natural killer cells).

When your immune system weakens, it no longer has the resources to keep its defences in optimal condition and slowly over time you may develop immune system issues: allergies, immune deficiencies and autoimmune disorders. Eat badly, sleep poorly, skip the exercise and your immune system will struggle to protect you as it should.

Fever: developing a high temperature is the body's way of killing off disease. It sends a signal that mobilises the entire immune system to work harder to fend off the viruses and begin to repair any damage they have done.

Immunity

This is a term that refers to your ability to be able to resist attack, whether from a virus, a bacteria, fungi or parasite. You develop immunity either by having been infected by a virus and having developed anti-bodies to it, or by being vaccinated against it.

Vaccines: These are a man-made method of duplicating the body's natural immune response. A vaccine is a laboratory created and treated virus, toxin or bacteria, usually injected into the body, triggering it to make new antibodies to a substance that it doesn't recognise.[1]

Herd Immunity: When a large percentage of the population have been vaccinated against an infection, and/or another large percentage have had the disease and developed antibodies against it, all those people will have immunity against a virus and the progression of the disease amongst the general population slows and is easier to manage.[2]

The problem with viruses:

The reason many people fall sick repeatedly, with the common cold or flu, for example, is that viruses mutate rapidly, developing slightly different strains of the same type of virus. Although you may have developed immunity against the original type, you won't have it against these new variations. Vaccines are developed based on past years information, which is why you may have a current winter flu jab and yet still fall sick with the flu. The virus moved quicker than the science!

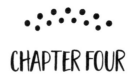

CHAPTER FOUR

IMMUNE SYSTEM ACTION PLAN

The Three Keys

In the absence of vaccines and effective anti-viral drugs, it makes sense to look to nature for help to work alongside conventional medical solutions. For thousands of years, plant and mineral remedies have been shown to work against viral infection. There is currently little science available to show results with COVID-19, but that is because the virus has only recently emerged, and research takes years to complete. There are, however, evidence-based studies on a multitude of other viruses, many of them also versions of the coronavirus, and that research is well worth knowing about.

Nature has given us a tool kit for most eventualities – it is up to us to learn about and use it.

There are three keys to improving the strength of your immune system

1. Establish how its currently working

2. Unload anything that could weaken it

3. Boost it

The First Key: Establish the strength of your immune System

Science has developed comprehensive in-depth tests that can look at every aspect of your immune health, examining natural killer cell counts and overall function. Mobilising stem cells and immune cells for cryo storage, for example, will raise natural killer cells count up to 14 times their normal levels. These techniques, however, are not available to the majority of us, so its vital to find alternatives that will give you a clear idea of what in your body is not working as it should, and identify ways to optimise recovery.

The Ogden Home Health Solution Kit Developed by a naturopathic doctor, this provides an immediate, 'do at home' way of monitoring your immune system, allowing you to track how it changes over a period of time. Viruses thrive in an acid environment, and on high sugar and low oxygenation. This kit allows you – and four other family members - to test a wide range of key functions. It contains a glucose meter and glucose strips, cholesterol meter and strips, saliva pH testing strips, a urine dipstick test, a blood pressure meter, a temperature gun, pre-injection swabs, and a digital blood oxygenation meter. The kit is particularly useful for people with underlying health issues such as those with:

Diabetes - Glucose shows your sugar levels. Do you know if you are pre-diabetic?

Cardiovascular disease – Cholesterol is a marker for cardiovascular disease

Chronic respiratory illness – SpO2 (Blood oxygenation) and Peak Flow show the condition of your lungs and whether you are breathing correctly – or not.

High blood pressure – this should be regularly monitored.

It comes with instructions on how to improve any markers that are currently out of range. There is also an online phone call booking system for individualised advice. (contact: johnogden11@gmail.com)

Health Baseline Testing: Essential for tracking whether your health is improving or deteriorating, my book, *'Reboot your Health: Simple DIY Tests and Solutions to Assess and Improve Your Health'* offers inexpensive easy to do tests, followed up with natural remedies and other answers – available on Amazon £12.99 and on my website www.reboothealth.co.uk.

The Second Key: Unload what weakens your immune system

Spending a longer amount of time at home than normal gives you the chance to pay attention to the finer details of your health. Grasp these days as an opportunity to re-organise your life. It's as important to find out what might be affecting and weakening your immune system as it is to making it stronger. And often positive immunity boosting strategies won't be as effective as they should be if you haven't dealt with the underlying issues first. There are four areas to start with:

Toxic metals

Metals are toxic to the human body. They can trigger thyroid dysfunction, inflammation, hormonal problems, bloating and stomach issues. They weaken the immune system and lower your natural defences, which is the last thing you need in times of viral infection. You can breathe metals in from the air, take them in from water and even the pans you cook with can add to your load. Cadmium, lead and aluminium are linked to Parkinson's, Alzheimer's and dementia. Studies of various cancer groups also showed that aluminium and cadmium levels were elevated in all patients. Mercury in your teeth can damage both the heart and the central nervous system.[1]

Action Plan

Send off for a Hair Mineral Analysis test: Post off a few small samples of hair from your head to a lab to be tested for toxic metals and mineral deficiencies. Once you receive the initial report you can then work towards correcting it. You will get back around 11 pages of analysis, listing your levels of chromium, molybdenum, sulphur, zinc and potassium, mercury, copper, cadmium, lead and arsenic. (biolab.com)

Do a metal detox: My book – '*Get Wise, Get Well*', available on Amazon, explains in detail how to remove metals from your body naturally and with no side effects. Or consult a naturopathic doctor or herbalist for a detox programme.

Drink silica rich Acilis water: Aluminium is a powerful immunosuppressant, so removing it from your body can only be beneficial. In clinical trials involving both healthy individuals and individuals with disease, drinking around a litre of silicon-rich mineral water every day was found to speed up the removal of toxic aluminium from the body via the kidneys and ultimately urine. Participants found 'significant reductions in their body burden of aluminium, including falls of up to 70% in one case, over a 12-week period'.[2]

Mould

Mould is rarely on your doctors list of possible triggers for illness and it doesn't show up in blood tests. Very few people think of mould as a threat, yet it is one of the most dangerous toxins you can be exposed to, and, according to the World Health Organisation, dampness and mould are estimated to affect 10-50% of homes in Europe, North America, Australia, India and Japan. In the US, the figures are particularly high, at approximately 50 - 80%.

Dr Richard Shoemaker, who has studied the effects of mould on thousands of patients, has concluded that fungal toxins cause chronic inflammation in the body, paralysing the systems that would usually control it. The body's protective mechanisms stop working, and the immune system begins to fail. Alzheimer's, ADHD, autism, behavioural problems, as well as heart attacks, have all been linked to the effects of mycotoxins. Chronic fatigue, fibromyalgia and Lyme's Disease have been shown to have a connection to mould too. Brain fog, depression, joint pain, pneumonia, weight gain, sinus infection, sore throats: the list goes on and on.

Action Plan

Take a mould test: The Visual Contrast Sensitivity Test measures how well you see details and contrast, and a poor result may indicate a mould issue. (VCSTest.com) Or check out www.irlen.com and take their light sensitivity test. When you are affected by mould, you become extra sensitive to light and sound.

Read my book: '*The Mould Menace: Fix Your Body, Fix Your Mind*' is a comprehensive overview of all mycotoxin related issues. It tells you what to look out for and how to go about resolving any problems. Cleaning up the mould in your home could well improve the strength of your immune system. Be careful how you go about it though, and understand the topic in greater detail before you attempt a clean-up. Available on Amazon.

Chemical Overload

So many new and unnatural substances have been created in the last few decades that we are bombarded by 1,000s of chemical toxins every day. Our food is no longer safe from genetic modification (GMO) and chemical interference. Synthetic fertilisers and pesticides are making the Earth – and ourselves – sick. In addition, our homes are built with products known to be carcinogenic – including lead, PVC, creosote, flame-retardant chemicals, and the volatile organic compounds (VOCs) found in solvents, paints and plastic coatings.

We then fill our homes with furniture made from similarly harmful cleaning products and toiletries, make-up, hair spray, sun creams, body lotions, perfume, and shower and bath gels. We breathe them in and rub them into our skin. Over time they build up in the body, hampering its ability to rid itself of the unwanted synthetic chemical by-products. Residues from plastics in bottles, pesticides and detergents are an obvious example – they mimic hormones, blocking oestrogen or progesterone and wreak havoc with your body and brain.

They weaken your immune system.

Action Plan

Make a list of toxins that you come into contact with day-to-day:

Look at the products you use in the bathroom: Read the labels on your toothpaste and your shampoos; If you can't understand what it says, it is not likely to be a natural substance. Do the same for the products under your kitchen sink, or in the cleaning cupboard. However much or little you lighten the chemical load will make a difference to your immune system.

Swop to organic: As you use up your current products, consider buying organic the next time round. Your lungs in particular will breathe more easy!

Parasites

We all have parasites living in our gut, and most are caught from undercooked meats, unwashed vegetables and fruits or contaminated water and foods. There are thousands of different types of parasites and the only way to test for them reliably is via your doctor or nutritionist. While you are spending more time inside, this is the perfect time to lighten your parasitic load, which will similarly lighten your immune systems load dealing with them. Wash your hands often. You are more likely to be subject to infection from parasites when your immune system is weak, and people are particularly vulnerable whilst undergoing treatment for cancer, or long-term, or chronic conditions such as HIV.

Action Plan

Start taking anti-parasite supplements daily. Your natural health store will have a range of traditional botanical formulas that have historically been used against parasites. The ayurvedic remedy Mimosa pudica powder destroys parasites over a 3-month period. Take 1/2 teaspoon twice a day, twice a week initially increasing to a teaspoon a day.

Cook with more anti-parasite foods and spices: eat more garlic, chilli, turmeric, thyme and ginger.

Up your pet hygiene: Pets, particularly dogs and cats, may play host to highly contagious roundworms that can migrate to humans. Wash your hands after stroking them, and prevent them from licking your face and lips. Don't let them anywhere near your dishwasher and plates!

 The Third Key: Boost Your Immune System

Build up your 'good' gut bacteria

When your immune system is weakened by a viral overload, often it is your lungs and your gut that are heavily compromised.

There are estimated to be a flabbergasting 100 trillion microbes living alongside and inside you. As a group, microbes are described as your 'microbiota' and the term 'microbiome' refers to your own personal microbe ecosystem – made up of individual varieties and quantities of microbe types specific to you.

Your body has 3 times more bacterial cells than human cells. And as viruses alone outnumber bacteria in the human gut 5 to 1, the size and power of your microbiome is truly galactic - comparable in numbers, literally, to the stars and planets of outer space.[3]

Only around 1,000 microbes have been identified in humans, and the same ones pop up time and time again. On average each individual will have a combination of around 160 bacteria making up his microbiome and each area of the body has different inhabitants adapted for that particular environment. Skin microbes tend to be similar in all of us, but very different, for example, to the microbes found in the gut.

Take probiotics: A healthy diet, backed up by supplementing with pro-biotics and adding fibre for them to feed on and increase their numbers, is an effective way of protecting the gut from viral attack. Probiotics have repeatedly been shown to stimulate – and equally importantly, to modulate - the immune system and certain strains have been found to be effective anti-virals.

If you are looking for a good all-round immune system boosting probiotic, then right now, based on what you can buy in the shops, Lactobacillus and Bifidobacterium are the names to choose. Higher numbers are better, so look for a count of 50 billion or higher in each dose. Choose a product with as many different strains as possible but more is not necessarily better than a few strategically targeted strains, so check on the web for information about research into probiotics that might works for your health issue.

If you are currently on a course of antibiotics, or have taken some recently, it is vital to restock your gut microbiome to protect yourself against viral infection. Taking a course of antibiotics is very similar to setting off a bomb inside your gut. They wipe out everything, good and bad bacteria included, though unfortunately not the viruses themselves, so make sure you take probiotics during (at a different time of day) and afterwards, and eat sensibly to reseed your gut for several weeks afterwards. Supplement with prebiotics to feed them and give them the strength they need to recolonise.

Effective anti-viral probiotics for lung and gut

Specific strains have been shown to be helpful for lung issues which are frequently associated with viral infection[4]. Most probiotics can affect respiratory viruses by triggering changes to your immune system responses. They have been shown to prevent viral and bacterial infections in the intestines, the urogenital tract and the lungs. They reduce acidity levels in the body and can produce additional levels of vitamins B and C. Scientists have now developed a specific term for them – 'immunobiotics'.

Lactobacillus acidophilus has been shown to activate NK cells in the lungs[5] and combined with B Bifidum it reduced respiratory tract infection symptoms in school children who contracted a viral infection and led to a decrease in absence from school.

Lactobacillus plantarum has been shown to successfully suppress viral proliferation in the lungs in a study of H1N1 infection[6]. In a study carried out on mice infected with pneumovirus, it increased their survival rates and reduced inflammatory response.[7]

Lactobacillus rhamnosus helps with diarrohea and triggers an anti-viral respiratory immune response[8]. The L. rhamnosus LGG strain decreases the severity of symptoms and length of illness in respiratory tract infections.

continued...

Lactobacillus reuteri reduces inflammatory response linked to pneumovirus[9]

Lactobacillus fermentum has been shown to boost immune response, increase antibodies and nitric oxide production in a study of the H1N1 virus.[10] In another study it was shown to reduce the number and length of upper respiratory tract infections.[11]

Lactobacillus casei decreased the length of the illness period of respiratory tract infections by a day. [12]

Bifidobacterium longum - shown in a study of H1N1 to lead to a decrease in symptoms and prevent body weightloss.

Take Biobran

Biobran has been shown to dramatically boost levels of white blood cells and raise NK (natural killer cell) levels more than 35 times in the space of four weeks. Developed more than 20 years ago in Japan, Biobran is a natural supplement made from rice bran broken down by the enzymes of Shitake mushrooms. It comes as a single daily pill which releases its powerful contents first into your small intestine and then on into your blood, where it activates those vital immune cells and triggers cell death in cancer cells. Within two to three weeks, NK cell levels have been shown to increase by up to 300%, B-cells by 250% and T-cell numbers by 200%. And all without side effects of any kind.

Dr Ghoneum of Charles Drew University of Medicine and Science in Los Angeles has described it as the most powerful immune booster he has ever found. Biobran is not meant to be a replacement for conventional medical treatment, but helps to support it, working hand in hand with pharmaceutical solutions to raise your numbers of NK cells and T and B cells to optimal levels.

There are currently 43 published peer reviewed papers on Biobran demonstrating how it works. It has been shown to help rheumatoid arthritis, virally triggered ME, Hepatitis B & C, HIV and diabetes as well as cancer. Biobran reduces inflammation throughout the body as well as reducing the side effects of chemotherapy. Recent trials show it can also successfully control and clear the HPV virus connected to cervical cancer. [13] Available from The Really Healthy Company – www.healthy.co.uk

Add wheatgrass to your daily diet

Wheatgrass is 70% chlorophyll, and has been described as the plant kingdoms 'blood equivalent', almost structurally identical to our own blood's haemoglobin. Chlorophyll wipes out bacteria, removes toxins and boosts your tired liver. Drinking freshly juiced wheatgrass energizes your tissues, raises your enzyme levels and speeds up your metabolism. It is said to reduce high blood pressure and improve circulation.

Chlorophyll is also a blood purifier, and wheatgrass will detox your organs faster than most other options.

It contains high levels of vitamins A, C, D, K and the B complexes, as well as B17, the cancer fighting Laetrile. A tiny glass of wheatgrass apparently contains more than 100 minerals and vitamins. It is high in oxygen, allowing both your body and brain to thrive. Drink a small shot daily and you multiply and re-energise both your red and your white blood cells and rapidly reboot the immune system, balancing your blood sugar in the process.

You can buy it in freeze dried capsule form or frozen, but as ever fresh is best. Producers can deliver boxes to your door. Put it through your juicer and drink within a few minutes or the nourishment dissipates and disappears. Experiment with a couple of 2oz shots a day and track your energy levels over the period of a week.

> **Top Tip:** Aconbury Sprouts on www.wheatgrass-uk.com will deliver wheatgrass direct to your door for around £5 a tray. They also sell frozen wheatgrass.

Colloidal Silver

You can buy this in most health stores. Spray it up each nostril and to the back of your throat for anti-viral protection. Colloidal silver's ability to destroy even the microbes that are most resistant to the strongest antibiotics has been repeatedly scientifically proven. In the 1980s, at UCLA medical school, Larry C. Ford, MD, documented over 650 different disease-causing pathogens, including viruses, that were destroyed in minutes when exposed to small amounts of silver. A 2015 study found colloidal silver was 'highly effective' in the treatment of MRSA, the flesh-eating, anti-biotic resistant bacteria frequently found in hospitals.[14] A separate laboratory test carried out on a group of silver based products compared each one's ability to kill MRSA, and found that Altrient's ACS 200 killed 99.999955% of the microbes. It was found to be 4,000 times more effective than the others, killing over 20 million MRSA organisms within 2 minutes.[15]

Colloidal Silver works for sinusitis, colds, flu, bronchitis and even pneumonia. Use a nebulizer to get it deep into your lungs. Never use it for more than about 10 days in a row, and supplement with a good probiotic, so you replace the bacteria it's destroying with ones that will boost your system. Supplement with selenium additionally to minimise any adverse reactions. Combine with curcumin to destroy the biofilm where the viruses hide, that protects them from being 'seen' and destroyed by your immune system. It is anti-inflammatory and provides a powerful boost for your immune system. Tiny nanoparticles in hydrosol silver are reputed to be more potent than colloidal or other types of silver.

Get Thymus Tapping

The thymus gland, which sits in the centre of your chest just above your heart and about 1.5 inches below the notch in your sternum, plays a major part in immunity and keeping you healthy. It pumps out white blood cells, acting as an incubator for disease fighting T-cells. It is at its largest in childhood and starts shrinking after puberty, so that by your mid 50's you will have about 15% left, and by the time you get to your early 70's it may have disappeared altogether. Loss of its function makes you more susceptible to viral attack but you can boost it and strengthen your immune system by tapping on the point above your thymus. Tap with the four fingers of your right hand, for about 20 seconds daily, to stimulate it, and keep it awake and working.[16]

Alkalise your body

Stress creates acidity and viruses thrive in an acid environment. The more anxious you are, therefore, the more vulnerable you become. Balance your mental stress by strengthening the physical. Get alkalising your body and start by cutting out sugar, flour and processed foods. Add raw foods, vegetables and green juices into your diet. Flooding your cells with alkaline foods can balance your pH, and decrease inflammation. And apple cider vinegar is the queen of alkalising tonics. Throat acidity makes you more vulnerable to viral and bacterial infections, so pour two tablespoons - of the cloudy version - into a mug of warm water and sip slowly. (See gargling p 83)[17]

Eat an Anti-viral Diet

Eat organic fresh fruit and vegetables as often as you can and cut down on sugar and processed junk food. Ideally, each of us should be having 5 servings a day for optimal health. A multitude of studies have shown that this can reduce the risk of a stroke by 26% and decrease your chance of dying from cardiovascular disease by a remarkable 49%. Plant flavonoids help boost antioxidants and reduce free radicals, boosting the immune system. They are also anti-inflammatory and anti-viral.[18]

Add in:

Bananas: Research shows that the high levels of potassium in bananas supports lung function and may be associated with lower risk of wheezing in childhood asthma. They also help the lungs to contract and expand more easily which could be useful for breathing problems associated with viral infection. Their natural fibre also provides food for your gut 'good' bacteria – a natural 'pre-biotic'.[19]

Enzyme rich green vegetables: Fresh, organic, raw, leafy greens are full of enzymes, the magic bullets you need for a whole-body reboot. If you eat too many enzyme-less processed foods your digestive system stops working properly. It eventually weakens, leaving you more vulnerable to infection. Add kale, lettuce, cucumbers, sugar snap peas, sprouted seeds and herbs to your diet. Anything green, alive and full of chloryphyll transfers that living energy to your body.

Juices: If you can't quite face the thought of all those bowls of vegetables and plates of salad, then juicing may well be your easy answer. To optimise the health benefits of a daily juice, follow the 20-minute rule. Make it yourself, and drink it immediately, when all the enzymes, vitamins and other phyto-nutrients are at 100%.

Sweet Basil (Ocimum basilicum): This is the basil with dark leaves. Research has shown that it is an effective anti-viral, preventing, for example, the cocksackievirus from replicating post infection. It acts similarly for enterovirus, also reducing the possibility of getting an infection in the first place. Add to your salads daily.[20]

Fermented foods: Fermented foods encourage the growth of the 'good' bacteria in your gut, and when their levels are high, so are your immune levels, defending you from viral infections that might lay you low. Try a daily spoonful or two of sauerkraut, miso or kefir.

Anti-viral chicken soup

Dr Stephen Rennard of the University of Nebraska Medical Center carried out laboratory tests to understand why chicken soup had developed a world-wide reputation for rapid recovery from upper respiratory tract infections and colds and flu. The blood samples he examined showed that the soup reduced the movement of neutrophils, the white blood cells that defend the lungs against infection and which cluster to the surfaces of the airways, triggering coughs and sputum. The chicken and the vegetables in the soup also had anti-inflammatory effects which further relieved symptoms.

Dr Rennard's 'Grandma's Chicken Soup' recipe

Ingredients
- 5-6lb chicken
- 3 large onions
- 1 large sweet potato
- 3 parsnips
- 2 turnips
- 11 to 12 large carrots
- 5 to 6 celery stems
- 1 bunch of parsley
- salt and pepper to taste

continued...

Clean the chicken, put it in a large pot, and cover it with cold water. Bring the water to the boil. Add the onions, sweet potato, parsnips, turnips, and carrots. Boil about 1.5 hrs. Remove fat from the surface as it accumulates. Add the parsley and celery. Cook the mixture about 45 min longer. Remove the chicken. The chicken is not used further for the soup. Put the vegetables in a food processor until they are chopped fine or pass through a strainer. Salt and pepper to taste. [21]

Curcumin: Curcurmin is effective against both bacteria and viruses, successfully wiping out the HIV virus[22], Herpes simplex virus, Hepatitis C and the flu virus. It has had similar success with HPV[23], Zika virus[24] and Chikungunya virus[25] and is also a potent anti-inflammatory[26].

Ginger: Ginger contains high levels of iron, zinc, calcium and magnesium, and is a powerful anti-viral. Fresh ginger strengthens your respiratory system, dry ginger does not. Excellent for colds, flu, chest infections and sore throats.[27]

Garlic: Garlic is a potent anti-viral, and eating it raw, or as a liquidised (uncooked) puree alongside your normal food, will wipe-out certain flu and cold viruses though there is no current evidence that it can help prevent or tread COVID-19. In nature, one of garlics main components, allicin, is what protects the garlic bulb from attack by any microbes in the soil. Supplementing with allicin stimulates immune cells, kills pathogens and detoxifies carcinogens, boosting your immune system to help protect you from viral infection.

> **Top Tip:** Allitech Liquid is 100% allicin and is said to destroy most viruses in under a month. Take 2 teaspoons a day (dulwichhealth.co.uk).

Apples: Apples have been shown to slow decline in lung function. They decrease oxidative stress and keep inflammation in check which will also help your lungs remain stronger.[28]

Take out:

Grains with gluten: Eating too much bread, pasta and processed food triggers inflammation in the gut and lungs. Try the supermarket gluten free ranges or cut out altogether.

Dairy: Milk products thicken the production of mucous in the lungs. As the COVID-19 virus attacks the lungs, anything you can do to clear and strengthen them will hopefully minimise the severity of any symptoms.

Saturated Fats: Reduce the amount of meat, eggs and dairy that you eat. Research shows that higher levels correlate to higher levels of progression of infection of the HIV virus. As cholesterol levels went down, so too did the replication of the HIV-1 viral particles.[29]

Alcohol: Alcohol decreases the numbers of your gut bacteria leaving you with a weaker shield against any virus. Cut out drinking beer, wine and particularly spirits such as gin or vodka.

CHAPTER FIVE

SLEEP ACTION PLAN

Proper, deep sleep can boost your immune system. It is a crucial tool in the fight against viruses and infections, so take the time to help yourself sleep better. When you sleep, your body releases important proteins, antibodies and immune cells, all of which help to fight infections and inflammation.

How long should you sleep?

There is no such thing as the right amount of sleep. Everybody is different, with most people needing between 6 to 8 hours a night. Recent research seems to indicate that around seven hours is optimal, although this is hotly debated. However, experts agree that sleep quality is what counts, and in order to measure it, it's important to consider more than just the number of hours spent asleep.

As well as impacting on your health in countless ways, your sleep quality is also a barometer for your state of mind and wellbeing.

Keep a Sleep Diary

There are two main types of sleep problem: not being able to get to sleep in the first place, and waking up in the night (often several times) and struggling to get back to sleep.

Over the course of three nights, spaced out over a week or so, keep a notebook by your bed and track how you slept the night before. First thing in the morning, make a note of the following:

1. Estimated time it took you to get to sleep

2. Number of hours between falling asleep and waking up (how much sleep you've had)

3. Did you wake up in the night? If so, at what time, and how often, and how easily did you get back to sleep?

4. Any dreams or nightmares?

5. Did you wake up naturally, or artificially (ie. alarm)?

6. How did you feel when you woke up?

Keeping a note of your sleep state now and comparing it in a few weeks' time is a helpful marker of your progress.

Action Plan

Get yourself into a steady bedtime routine: Go to bed at the same time each night and regulate your body clock. Before 10.30pm is best because the hours before midnight are the body's most efficient fix and repair time. After that your adrenals kick in with a 'staying up late' boost of adrenaline, making it that much harder to sink in to a deep restorative sleep.

Cut down on coffee: Give it up altogether if you can, but otherwise, limit yourself to a cup or two before 11am in the morning. Did you know that just like uranium, coffee also has a half-life? Luckily, at only 5 hrs, it's a short one compared to the expiry of toxic radioactive substances, but that still means that 50% of the caffeine in your afternoon cup is still keeping you wide awake when you want to be winding down. Drink a cup after supper and your chances of sleeping deeply are minimal.

Exercise more: Exercise decreases your stress hormones and helps to boost mood and calm your mind. When you exercise, you sleep better. (See chapter six)

Read Up on Natural Sleep Remedies: My book *'Reboot Your Sleep'*, available on Amazon, offers a comprehensive overview of top tips to get you sleeping solidly throughout the night.

Bedroom Basics: It sounds obvious, but we all spend so much time in our rooms, watching TV, working on the computer, playing on laptops and ipad's and texting on our phones, that the bedroom is rarely synonymous with sleep. For your brain to relax deeply, remove all stimulants. Take out any electronics, including your bedside clock or radio. If you are supersensitive, even a plug socket too close to your head can affect your rest. If your bedroom is too hot your body will struggle to sleep throughout the night: too noisy, and you will wake frequently throughout the small hours. Consider investing in a white noise machine, or a small fan, to drown out any external sounds.

Black it out: Make sure your room is entirely dark. Bright light stimulates the pineal gland in the brain, creating serotonin, which keeps you happy and wakeful. Darkness on the other hand triggers melatonin, which makes you sleepy. Put in blackout blinds if you need to.

Pre-bed sleep habits

Do the same thing every night before you go to sleep. Just like letting a baby know that it is night time by following the same routine at the same time each evening, do the same thing for your mind.

Have a warm bath with sleep inducing lavender oils, listen to the same music, lie in bed and do a relaxation exercise. Hot baths help you sleep because your body has to drop its core temperature to get rid of the excess heat from the water, and that makes you drowsy.

Oddly, doing exactly the opposite may also work for you. Having a coldish shower before bed can also help you drift off to sleep. That also cools the core temperature and it's easier to sleep in the cold (look at bears and tortoises who hibernate in the winter). Cold lowers your heart rate and blood pressure, sending a message to your nervous system that it's time to relax and sleep.

Experiment: See if hot or cold at night works best for you.

6 Quick fix sleep techniques

Make yourself a cup of Valerian tea – Valerian is Nature's Valium. It should help you drift off in a matter of minutes

Get deep breathing: Try placing your hand on your stomach and breathe in deeply, so that your stomach rises. Spend a minute or two focusing on how it moves up and down as you breathe steadily and calmly in and out. Inhale for 3 seconds and then exhale for 5. Whenever your mind starts to drift away and think about other things, bring it firmly back to those rhythmic movements and you will find yourself asleep before you know it. Usually in less than a minute.

Invest in a magnesium oil spray, and spray it liberally on your arms and legs before you get into bed. (Allow it to soak in first or it will stain your sheets!). Magnesium is excellent for sleep and the oil penetrates rapidly into your bloodstream; far faster as a remedy than swallowing it in pill or capsule form.

Open the window or turn off the radiator. Cool is best, because your body releases melatonin at lower temperatures – ideally between 16-18˚C. Cold lowers your heart rate and blood pressure sending a message to your nervous system that it's time to sleep. Too hot a room temperature, however, and your body won't rest.

The Castor Oil pack: Try rubbing castor oil on to the area of skin above your liver, under the ribs of your right-hand side. Put a hot water bottle on top and lie back and relax.

Eat two kiwi fruits before bed! A recent study found that eating a couple of kiwi fruit an hour before bed improved both length and depth of sleep.[1]

What NOT to do if you can't sleep

Don't lie awake worrying, with your thoughts racing round your head repeatedly. Always have a notebook by the side of your bed, and write them down, turning them into a 'Tomorrows To-Do list'. The act of physically transferring them onto paper seems to give your brain the message – 'OK – tick. Got the message – will be deal with in the morning'. That seems to be sufficient – it frees your brain from the responsibility of needing to keep bringing the issues to your attention and you can drift off to sleep once more, unburdened.

Don't grab yourself a glass of wine, hoping it will make you comatose. It may briefly achieve its object, but alcohol is a stimulant, and after the initial drowsy response, you will find yourself even more wired than before.

Don't turn the light on and start reading your ipad or a book. All you will do is upset the circadian rhythms that are meant to keep you in a state of deep sleep in the middle of the night, making your brain think its morning instead.

CHAPTER SIX

EXERCISE ACTION PLAN

If you are lying in bed suffering from a viral infection, it is unlikely that exercise will be foremost in your mind. But if you are self-isolating, quarantined or recovering, exercise is a potent anti-viral defence. And if you aren't, a packed gym class with equipment used by hundreds of people is probably not the place to be. Swop to exercising outside where you can and otherwise use the latest technology to bring the gym into your living room. Move more and your immune system will strengthen. It's that simple.

Why you need to exercise

Exercising for anti-viral benefits is all about oxygen. When you exercise, you increase your circulation (the rate at which blood is pumped around your body). When your circulation increases, your blood can deliver more oxygen and more nutrients to your cells and tissues helping them stay fit and healthy, upping your energy levels, getting rid of toxins and keeping your body's systems working efficiently, both defending against viral attack and disposing of the viruses more efficiently.

It is also suggested that the rise in body temperature that is associated with exercise makes it harder for bacteria and viruses to thrive.

As you increase your breathing rate too, you flush your lungs and your airways out a bit more and therefore get rid of bacteria and viruses quicker.

For one person, a brisk walk might qualify as moderate-intensity exercise. For others, it's going to be an uphill sprint on a bike. It's about doing what's right for you.

You know you are doing moderate-intensity exercise if you are getting slightly out of breath when you are exercising. This, of course, means different things to different people. You should still be able to talk, but not sing. If you can sing you could probably be doing a bit more. If you can't even talk, you are probably working too hard!

The key to cardiovascular exercises is rhythmic movement of the limbs and the subsequent increase in the heart rate. That's what boosts the circulation and helps the immune system to function to the best of its capability.

How to get your muscles moving

Regular walking at a steady fast pace is excellent if you can go outside. If you are housebound, set yourself an increasing number of stairclimbing sessions, or choose an exercise YouTube video.

Book out a daily half hour for stretching, which is easy to do at home and necessary to keep your limbs supple, and your muscles and joints flexible. Add in yoga or Pilates or a gentle stretching class to release tension. If you stretch at home, always ease slowly into each position, and hold for 20 seconds or so before releasing gently, breathing steadily throughout. Never make any sharp movements that might stress your body.

High Intensity Interval Training

HIIT can help rapidly boost your energy levels and recovery. In a study at the Mayo clinic, over 65s who started a HIIT regime saw age-related deterioration in muscle cells reduced, and research published in 'Cell Metabolism' found levels of mitochondria, the cells energy powerhouses, increased considerably after a three-month HIIT programme. There was 49% more mitochondrial capacity in younger participants, and a 69% increase in older people.[1] HIIT training has also been found to be a better way to combat central obesity.

I do see the logic of interspersing fast-paced maximum-effort intervals of exercise with slower recovery periods. I just don't like doing it much. Take it very easy and build up over time. My version of HIIT, which is admittedly less strenuous than most people's, involves similarly short bursts of intense exercise - for 20 seconds at a time followed by a 10 second rest, repeated 5 times. Simple - and in total shouldn't take up much more than a few short minutes. Lose weight, burn off some fat and, according to research in the Journal of Sports Science, stimulate your human growth hormone levels, increasing them by 450%. Depending on your stage of recovery it is best to double check with your doctor before you start.[2]

My Mini HIIT circuit

This can be applied to any cardiovascular activity-walking/ cycling/rowing/running or swimming. Not advised if you have heart problems. Check with your doctor to minimise risk of any injury.

- Choose your activity and start by warming up with five minutes of light exertion.
- Standing tall, circle your arms backwards, one after the other for 30 seconds.
- Then up the intensity of your chosen activity and really go for it for 30 seconds.
- Rest for ten seconds
- Do another 30 seconds at the higher intensity
- Rest for ten seconds
- Do another 20-30 seconds at high speed
- Rest for ten seconds, repeat twice more.
- Then cool down

Exercise in the Green: Exercising outdoors or looking at a green view has been proven to lower your blood pressure and makes you happier than walking along a tree-less, concrete city street. Even a plant in the office can help you take less sick days and increase office productivity.[3]

Online apps

There are a variety of online fitness apps, so you don't need to abandon your fitness regime. Take the gift of enforced time to up your core strength, and get your body back on track.

Three of the best:

Vidawellness: This is a member's only exercise programme and community aimed at older people, with a focus on keeping moving more easily, improving posture and feeling more confident as you age, keeping you active and healthy for longer. It offers more than 50 home exercise videos showing you how to improve your balance, strengthen your muscles or relieve stiff and aching joints. There's no joining fee and you pay £11 a month subscription. They are currently offering a 14-day free trial. Studio.vidawellness.co.uk

Obe offers more than 20 different classes, each one 28 minutes long and is offering a month's free trial for anyone in quarantine. It costs £22 a month and has three categories of exercise - Sweat, which covers dance, HIIT, cardio boxing and trampoline bouncing; Define, which is about building strength and toning, lengthening and sculpting your body, and Flow, which offers yoga and stretch classes. obefitness.com

Freeletics: Train with your own digital coach via an app. You can choose a male or female, and decide whether your goal is to get fit, get toned or lose weight. They ask you specific questions to rate your fitness levels before directing to you to the appropriate exercises. These are short, and targeted, and the more you train, the more it adapts to you. Freeletics.com

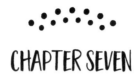

CHAPTER SEVEN

ANTI-VIRAL NUTRITIONAL SUPPLEMENTS

Many conventional doctors and health advisers say that there should be no need to supplement if you eat a balanced diet. However, modern lifestyles and eating habits, as well as a lack of nutrients in the soil due to modern farming practices and intensive pesticide use, mean that much of the food we eat is nutritionally depleted. Your immune system needs the full gamut of vitamins and minerals to keep it in optimal working order when it is under viral attack.

What to take and why?

Vitamin D

If you keep your Vitamin D levels high throughout the year your immune system should be able to fight off most viruses. Many of us, however, are low. Vitamin D is not something that can be made by the body. We get it in its natural form from sunlight on our skin, but living in Britain's grey and overcast land, there's not too much of that around for most of the year, and the majority of us are deficient. Do you know what your Vitamin D level is? Or even what it 'should' be? This may be one of the most important blood results you can ask for, and the NHS will now screen for it, free of charge, since the latest research has flagged its importance in immune function. The Vitamin D council suggests that a level of 50 ng/ml is the perfect level to aim for, and they recommend we all supplement with 5,000 iu daily to stay there. Vitamin D boosts immunity by increasing numbers of leukocytes, which are white blood cells that help defend against infectious diseases and unrecognised 'invaders'. Taking Vitamin K alongside (2 drops daily) will help increase the absorption of Vitamin D.

Zinc

Many of us are low in zinc, and yet it is needed by every cell in our bodies, and is a powerful immune booster. A potent anti-viral, zinc has been shown in a research study to inhibit the replication of coronavirus in cells.[1] Coronavirus affects the upper airways and respiratory disease is the major cause of illness and death with people infected with Covid-19 so supplementing with 11 mg of zinc daily may reduce susceptibility. Zinc deficiency is more common in elderly people who seem less able to absorb it – 20 mg per day was trialled in a French study of people in nursing homes which resulted in them experiencing less respiratory tract infections and having better antibody responses after the influenza vaccination than a control group who did not supplement with the mineral.[2]

Zinc acts directly in the throat, reducing the severity and duration of viral infection and so, if you suffer from respiratory symptoms, zinc pastilles may be an effective way to get your daily dose. 7 clinical trials in which participants took 6-10 slow dissolving (35 mins) zinc lozenges daily within the first few days of a cold found that both zinc gluconate and zinc acetate reduced the duration by an average of 33% compared to placebo.[3]

> **Top Tip:** Scientific theory suggests that zinc ions, when released into the upper respiratory system of a cold sufferer, interfere with the ability of the cold virus to reproduce. Cold-Eeze Homeopathic Cold Remedy (available in the USA) contains zinc gluconate – 12 mg and is the testing site consumerlab.com's top lozenge pick. Lamberts Zinc Plus lozenges release zinc, vitamin C and Bee Propolis to the throat membranes. Suck slowly over a 30 minute period and take 3-4 a day.

Vitamin A

Vitamin A protects the mucous membranes which is where the virus first takes hold. A daily dose of 800 mcg daily will make it harder for it to damage either your lungs or your gut.

Vitamin C

Your white blood cells – or leukocytes – are vital for helping your body fight off viral infection. There is no evidence that high doses of oral vitamin C can protect people from COVID-19 (mainly because there has been limited time since it was identified to carry these tests out) though currently high intravenous doses are being tested in patients in China.[4]

There is, however, solid evidence that Vitamin C boosts the immune system. It is a powerful anti-oxidant. Viruses thrive in an oxidised cellular environment and Vitamin C enhances antibody production, improving the function of the white blood cells that track down and destroy viruses and enhances anitbody production. It can also help in the fight against the viruses by increasing interferon production, released by virus infected cells to send messages to nearby cells to heighten their defences[5]. 1,000-2,000 mg a day as an anti-viral maintenance dose. If you develop symptoms take 1,000 mg every hour.

NAC

This is a powerful lung protector and should be taken by anyone with COPD or respiratory diseases of any kind. (600mg twice a day). It is an amino acid that helps to regenerate the damaged cells in the bronchi that occur with lower respiratory diseases. It is also a precursor for the endogenous antioxidant glutathione (antioxidants can be endogenous, made in the body – or exogenous, which means built-up by diet or dietary supplement). Take alongside selenium which enhances the body's uptake.[6]

Melatonin

This is a hormone with strong anti-inflammatory and immunity boosting effects. It has been shown to successfully destroy the influenza virus. This is the virus which can trigger an inflammatory response in the lungs that often leads to pneumonia. High levels of exposure to WiFi or electromagnetic fields has been shown to reduce melatonin levels. 50 mg or 2 drops 1-2 hrs before bed and 2-3 hrs after your last meal.[7]

Royal Jelly

Contains high concentrations of minerals, vitamins and anti-oxidants (1 dose daily). Honey and Royal Jelly when tested were both found to inhibit the growth of the Herpes simplex virus and reduce its numbers.[8]

My Daily Dose of Anti-viral Supplements

Vitamin D (at least 5000 IU daily)

Vitamin K2 (2 drops daily to support Vit D)

Vitamin C (2000 mg daily)

Zinc lozenges – 4 daily

Melatonin (2 drops before bed)

Essential oils – (I drop each of Thyme, Ravintsara and Oregano directly on the tongue daily)

continued...

NAC (2 each day – 1000mg in total optimal)

Royal Jelly (1 dose daily)

Oregano Oil – I capsule each morning

IV Therapy

What is an intravenous drip?

Intravenous (IV) Therapy or Intravenous Micronutrient Therapy (IVMT), is a treatment where a bag of carefully combined liquid nutrients, usually hanging on a tall metal stand, slowly drips its contents through a clear plastic tube into a canula inserted into a vein in your hand or arm. The nutrients pass rapidly into your bloodstream, where they are circulated around the body and used where they are wanted, by-passing the gastric juices that so often destroy vitamins and minerals that are swallowed down with a glass of water. Sessions usually take about an hour.

Why take your nutrients intravenously?

When you swallow a pill or capsule, it has to travel through the acidic digestive juices of the stomach, making its way through the small intestine, large intestine, the liver and then the blood vessels, absorbing through to the tissues and passing from the tissues to arrive at last where they are needed in the cell. Only a small percentage arrives at the final destination, with approximately 85% of the benefits lost on the journey. Taking those same nutrients intravenously gets them directly into the blood, and rapidly to whichever part of your body needs them, directly to the cells.

Scientific evidence

IV treatments have now been used as a medical tool for decades. Dr John Myers, after whom the popular Myers cocktail IV is named, incorporated it successfully in his Baltimore practise for years, and Dr Alan Gaby, from the same city, worked with more than 1,000 patients intravenously injecting them with liquid nutrients, eventually publishing his results in the 2002 Alternative Medicine Review (Vol 7, No 5).

Viral fighting IV's

Myers Cocktail

This is a combination drip that is frequently used in many IV clinics and is a great all-round booster. It includes essential vitamins and trace minerals – vitamin C, the B vitamins (B1,2,3,5,6,& B12), magnesium and folic acid, with different add-on's for specific nutritional boosts. It has been clinically trialled for fibromyalgia, with the results finding it entirely safe.[9]

Hydrogen Peroxide

Your cells need oxygen to survive and to carry out their daily tasks and Hydrogen Peroxide increases oxygen levels, helping to repair the body's tissues and boost white blood cells, reducing the plaque that builds up on the arteries and wiping out bacteria and viruses.

High Dose Vitamin C

Detoxs the body; speeds metabolism and supports the adrenals. Used as a cancer therapy and to neutralise bacteria and viruses. Reduces inflammation.

Vitamin B Complex – Minimises stress.

Sodium Bicarbonate

Liquid sodium bicarbonate alkalises your body's pH levels, wiping out bacteria and viruses in the process.

Curcumin

Reduces pain and inflammation and boosts immunity; anti-viral and speeds up recovery from chemo, boosting the liver and improving memory.

Silver Hydrosol

Pure silver in nano sized particles. Anti-microbial - used to treat bacterial, fungal and viral infections. Also offered for Lyme's disease.

DMSO

This is a sulfur compound that occurs in nature. It has anti-microbial, anti-fungal, and anti-viral properties. Boosts immunity and decreases susceptibility to infection.

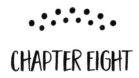

CHAPTER EIGHT

HARNESS THE POWER OF PLANTS

Stock up on essential oils

Viruses are hard to destroy because they surround themselves with a strong protein shell which forms an impenetrable shield around them. Essential oils, however, seem to be able to break through it. Each one contains anything from 80-750 natural variants of chemical components, which used in combination, can obliterate almost any virus, efficiently and thoroughly. Put them in a diffuser (3-5 drops) and breathe them in, add them to a glass of water, drop 2-3 drops into your bath water or add 1-2 drops to a carrier oil like coconut oil and rub directly on your skin to strengthen your immunity and ward off the microbes.

Each essential oil carries the entire essence of the plant it is taken from. The oil is the distillation of every bit of it – the leaves, the stem, the roots, the flowers or the bark. A natural pharmaceutical with healing power in a tiny bottle. The potency of a single drop of oil can equal several teaspoons of the plant in its dried form. I drop of peppermint, for instance, is the equivalent of more than 25 cups of peppermint tea. Make no mistake, essential oils are powerful. Tests have proven them to be anti-microbial, anti-viral, anti-inflammatory and anti-bacterial.

Top Tip: If you are using these oils against viral infection, give yourself a break after two weeks of continual use. Wait a few days before starting with them again.

Anti-viral essential oils

Eucalyptus - research indicates that this oil disrupts the virus' ability to penetrate cells walls. In a test against the H1N1 virus, the oil was 100% successful in destroying the pathogen within the space of 10 minutes.[1]

Oregano. A potent anti-viral. It is its ingredient, carvacrol, that is particularly effective at destroying the 'viral capsid', the protective sheath the virus is surrounded with. Another of its compounds, thymol, also has powerful antibacterial properties. A study in the journal 'Frontiers in Microbiology' found that a combination of oregano oil and silver nanoparticles was additionally effective.[2]

continued...

Cinnamon. Despite extensive testing, research scientist Dr. Jean Claude Lapraz has stated that he couldn't find any microbe that could survive in the presence of cinnamon or oregano essential oils. Research shows that cinnamon essential oil is particularly effective against flu viruses when combined with eucalyptus and rosemary essential oils.[3]

Clove. Eugenol, an active ingredient found in clove oil, seems to be able to damage the viruses envelope, de-activating their destructive ability and preventing them from replicating.[4]

Rosemary. Contains oleanolic acid which is particularly effective against influenza viruses. It works by de-activating the viral particles and weakening the protective shields that defend them.[5]

Star Anise. Star anise contains a powerful antiviral substance known as shikimic acid, which the pharmaceutical industry synthesises to create flu drugs.[6]

Thyme. Powerfully effective against viruses on its own, research has shown that combined with tea tree and eucalyptus oils, it can reduce viral infection by more than 96 percent.[7]

Sage. Found to be effective as a sanitiser and successful when pitted against the SARS virus which is a different form of coronavirus to the current COVID-19 version. Helps prevent acute respiratory symptoms.[8] **continued...**

Ravensara Aromatica is a powerful antiviral essential oil from Madagascar (don't confuse it with Ravintsara which is a species of cinnamonum camphora also from Madagascar but originally from China) that is therapeutically beneficial as an anti-viral, anti-bacterial and antiseptic oil. Helpful for respiratory or bronchial issues, it kills airborne viruses via a diffuser, and has been shown to successfully treat shingles, herpes and other viral based illnesses, easing pain and inflammation. **Ravintsara** is a gentler oil, containing high levels of 1,8-cineole which is particularly effective for respiratory or bronchial problems, also easing breathing when diffused.[9]

Essential oil cocktails:

On Guard oil: DoTerra's *On Guard*, is made up of a combination of clove bud, eucalyptus leaf, rosemary leaf and flower, cinnamon bark and leaf and wild orange peel. It smells of Christmas and not only boosts immunity, but it wards off and kills harmful bacteria and viruses.

I could only find one scientific test on this oil, and it was carried out on dogs not humans, but the researchers found that not only did *On Guard* weaken the flu virus that they were experimenting with but the oil prevented it from being able to replicate itself as strongly, making it easier for the immune system to overcome.

continued...

SOS Advance is a combination of essentials oils in a nano particle solution produced specifically to destroy bacteria and viruses on a cellular level. It boosts the immune system and detoxes the liver, kidneys, bladder and other organs as well as purifying the blood. It has a high pH which alkalises the body. (sosessentials.com)

Thieves oil: Young Living's virus and bacteria deterrent is their powerful Thieves Oil blend. Based on a 15th century recipe that combines clove, rosemary and other botanicals it is inspired by the tale of four French robbers who raided the houses and graves of plague victims, stealing jewellery and valuables, yet never succumbing to the dread disease. Eventually captured, they swopped torture (though they ended up on the gallows) for their secret recipe. Tests have proven the oil to successfully boost the immune system.

Plants: The Heavy Hitters
Astragalus

A powerful Chinese anti-viral herb used to boost immunity. Several studies have shown that it stimulates the immune system and is effective at combatting the common cold and influenza virus. Research has also shown that it inhibits the growth of the herpes simplex virus type 1.[10]

Cats Claw

A proven anti-viral, antibacterial and antifungal, Cat's Claw has been shown to be effective for viral infections, including shingles (herpes zoster), cold sores (herpes simplex) and AIDS (HIV) and increases immunity by approx. 60 percent. It stimulates the macrophages and granulocytes of the blood and controls production of lymphocytes.[11]

Elderberry

Viruses clad themselves in sharp spikes, using them, like hedgehogs, to protect themselves and then to attack and overrun your healthy cells. Watch under a microscope and you will see a virus attach itself to the smooth walls of your cell and stick its spikes through your cell membrane, allowing it first to gain a foothold, then to colonise and rapidly multiply.

Research has shown that protective compounds in the berries wipe out those viral spikes in a couple of days, preventing any further spreading. An Israeli study, looking at viruses and the efficacy of elderberry juice syrup, showed that those who took a daily dose recovered far quicker than the control group who didn't take anything at all. 20% were better within 24 hours, 70% in 48 hours, and 90% had recovered completely in 3 days. Elderberry extract inhibits the replication of human flu viruses, including strains of Influenza A and B, and H1N1, but no studies have to date been carried out on its efficacy against the new COVID-19.[12]

Nutritional experts suggest that primary use for COVID-19 should be as an immune system booster, and to stop taking it at the development of any symptoms.

Oregano oil

Oregano oil, made from the oil of the oregano plant, is a potent immune booster. In research it was found to be effective against respiratory viruses, such as the flu, and also salmonella. It's primary active component, carvacrol, is effective at destroying the outer shield – the capsid - of the viruses. Take a capsule a day, of wild oregano if possible.[13]

Coconut Oil

Only found in unrefined Virgin or extra virgin coconut oil that has not been refined, the compounds lauric acid and molaurin have been found to be effective virus combatants – though tests to date were on farm animals and on people with HIV. A research study on people with COVID-19 is currently in hand.[14]

Liquorice Root

A powerful antioxidant and immune stimulant, liquorice root has been confirmed as an effective anti-viral due to its high levels of triterpenoids and has the potential to become 'a novel broad-spectrum anti-viral medicine and will be widely used in clinical treatment....' A research study published in The Chinese Journal of Virology outlined its efficacy against the herpes virus, HIV, hepatitis and the influenza virus.

It was also found to be effective against the coronavirus infections SARS and MERS.2[15]

Echinacea

The jury has long been out about the efficacy of echinacea for the flu virus. Laboratory studies have shown that certain types of echinacea may be effective against coronaviruses, particularly products made from the leaves, flowers and stem of E. purpurea, dried and as a powder (900mg per day taken in 3 doses). It contains echinacein, a compound that prevents bacteria and viruses from penetrating healthy cells.

A laboratory study that has not yet been peer-reviewed found that a particular branded form of echinacea inhibited specific coronaviruses, including (HCoV) 229E, MERS- and SARS-CoVs, and the researchers suggested it could potentially have a similar effect on SARS-CoV-2, the coronavirus that causes COVID-19, although it was not tested.[16] As with elderberry, professionals suggest using it primarily as an immune booster and stopping if COVID -19 symptoms develop.

Andrographis (Andrographis paniculata) is a bitter tasting herb known as 'Indian echinacea', rich in compounds known as andrographolides which have anti-inflammatory, antiviral, and antioxidant properties. It has been found to reduce viral load and lung inflammation.[17]

Olive Leaf

A potent antiviral that is effective against the common cold and flu and virally triggered diseases such as meningitis, shingles, pneumonia, hepatitis B, malaria, gonorrhoea and tuberculosis. It contains compounds that stop the viruses reproducing themselves, destroying the outer shell that protects the microbes. The main compound is oleuropein, which is an antioxidant with antibacterial, anti-inflammatory and immune stimulating properties. Laboratory tests in a Saudi Arabian research project have shown that olive leaf is effective against herpes and rotavirus. It contains 400% of the anti-oxidants of vitamin C. The standard dose ranges from 500 mg to 1,000 mg daily, split into two or three separate doses. Do not take if you are on blood pressure drugs as it can cause your levels to fall; or if you are on insulin or chemotherapy. Please discuss with your doctor.[18]

Stevia

Stevia is made from the leaves of a small South American shrub and has proved itself an effective natural sugar sweetener, reducing calories, controlling diabetes and aiding weight management. It contains the compound stevioside which gives it its sweetness.[19]

A dried purified extract of Stevia was studied in laboratories, and successfully pitted against Teschen disease virus, infectious rhinotracheitis virus and human coronavirus.[20]

A research study from the University of New Haven found that exposing the bacteria B. burgdorferi to alcohol extracted stevia leaf permanently wiped out Lyme disease in all its different phases, including the hard-to-kill biofilm form. In a comparative control group, however, that was only treated with antibiotics, not only did the bacteria re-surface after approximately 7 days, but the numbers of bacteria protected by the biofilm multiplied exponentially.

Calendula

Marigold in its different forms has been used for medicinal purposes for centuries. It works against viruses and bacteria and protects against free radicals. It is available as a tincture, liquid, infusion, ointment or cream.[21]

Manuka Honey

Produced in New Zealand and famed for its medicinal powers, it has been shown to destroy antibiotic-resistant bugs. Opt for manuka with a 'UMF' of 10+ or more and eat a teaspoonful a day to ward off flu germs. 16 + is preferable.[22]

CHAPTER NINE

AIR, OZONE AND HEAT

Clean up your Air

One of the dangers of living in an environment where the windows are permanently closed is that the levels of pollutants continually rise – including the levels of bacteria and viruses. Higher levels of infection are often linked to places with sealed windows and air-conditioning with recycled air. Think cruise ships, offices, hospitals, hotels and blocks of flats with internal air circulation. The viruses have no way of being 'flushed out'. According to Christian Lickfett, air pollution expert & MD of Commercial Air Filtration, *'Indoor air, in all buildings…. can easily be ten times more polluted than outside air, as contamination is created and builds up in buildings'.*

If you can't get around this issue, and for whatever reason cannot get access to fresh air, invest in a diffuser and add anti-viral essential oils to the water (see p.68) which will keep any virus under control and eliminate build-up of numbers.

Action Plan

- Simply open your windows for a period first thing in the morning or later in the evening and disperse the indoor build-up of chemicals (just do it at times when air pollution is low).

- Invest in a Dyson Pure Cool air purifier which removes 99.95% of particles as small as 0.1 microns in the air inside your home. It automatically and continually monitors the indoor air quality in your rooms and adjusts the airflow accordingly. Once the air is improved it keeps it that way.

Oxygen Healing

Oxygen is vital to the health of our cells. It is turned into energy and used by the body for regeneration and repair and has been shown to prevent viruses from replicating. Increasing your oxygen levels is beneficial for your health. Tests have shown increased resistance to stress, and deeper sleep patterns.

Action Plan

- **Invest in an oxygen meter:** This is an inexpensive way of measuring how much - or how little - oxygen you have in your blood. It is a small clip that fits onto your finger and analyses both your blood oxygen saturation and your pulse and gives you a baseline reading going forward from which to aim to improve. Small, simple to use and reliable, doctors often use it to keep patients with lung and breathing issues stable. It gives you an early warning if your oxygen levels or pulse rate fall to a dangerous level. Available from Amazon.

- **Get your own personal oxygen system:** ClearO2 is an oxygen filled cannister that you can buy for less than £20. Keep one at home and boost your oxygen levels with a mere 8-10 inhalations a day. (clearO2.com)

- **Ask your doctor about a nebulizer:** This is an inexpensive machine that you can buy and use at home, infusing your lungs and brain with healing oxygen to up your anti-oxidant levels, and combining it with other substances that re-invigorate and repair. A clear plastic tube connects the nebulizer to a compressor which forces oxygen to flow at high speed through a liquid medicine, converting it into a fine mist that can then penetrate deep into your lungs. For people with lung problems - pneumonia, asthma, inflammation, emphysema or cystic fibrosis, - or even for coughs, colds and flu, a nebulizer is a painless way of getting medications deep into the lungs, easing the conditions and helping them to regenerate and heal at a rapid rate.

Scientific tests have shown that nebulization is just as effective as certain drugs, with the added benefit of no side effects. Adding glutathione reduces oxidative stress, decreases inflammation, and modulates T cell responses in the lungs. Magnesium, sodium bicarbonate, colloidal silver and hydrogen peroxide are all alternate nebulizing options for breathing problems.

What you are looking for if you google on the internet, are the inexpensive jet nebulizers priced usually between £30-£50 pounds. Then there are more expensive ultrasonic nebulizers that do the same thing only more silently. Beurer produce a good range, as does Omron. Your doctor will give you a prescription and precise dosage if you are suffering from a specific health issue.[1]

- **Hyperbaric oxygen treatment**, in a specially designed chamber, can weaken and destroy certain viruses. Breathing oxygen in through a nasal canula at pressure floods your bloodstream with pure oxygen, forcing oxygen deep into your body, where it is absorbed by your blood, liver, brain and all your cells and tissues, helping them to renew and repair.[2]

- **Vital Air Therapy:** Vital Air has developed a machine that improves the body's uptake and use of oxygen, improving the strength of the mitochondria, the cells 'energy batteries', and protecting the cells against the ravages of free radicals. It's website states that 'Vital Air Therapy is an Activated Oxygen Therapy which can help to relax the lungs and the cardio-vascular system, and improve the body's utilisation of oxygen by changing it into a more energised form, which is more readily usable by the body...' The company claims that it is helpful for asthma, COPD (chronic obstructive pulmonary disease), chronic bronchitis and emphysema. Vital-air-therapy.com

Oxidation

All diseases are linked to an increase in your oxidation levels, caused by the free radicals in your body. Pollution, radiation poor diet and lifestyle can increase these levels, triggering inflammation, premature ageing, and general physical degeneration. Normally your body produces 'anti-oxidants' as a protective measure to keep free radicals in check, but when your immune system is weak, it struggles to do this naturally. Upping levels of fruits and vegetables provides additional anti-oxidants that the body cannot produce on its own, restoring the natural balance and keeping damaging free radical numbers down.[3] Reduce your oxidation levels, and logically, your body will begin to recover.

Ozone

> **Warning:** *Direct exposure to ozone is not safe, particularly if you have an underlying health condition, so make sure that you – and any pets - are never in the room when you have your ozone generator switched on. Keep the windows closed and after switching it off, keep out of the room for a few hours, airing the space before you go back in.*

Ozone is a gas, made up of three atoms of oxygen but whilst oxygen is odourless, ozone has a strong distinctive smell and is harmful if breathed in for extensive periods. Its strength in times of infection is that it can be used to kill external bacteria and viruses on surfaces. Ozone breaks through the viral protective sheath, damaging its RNA and, at higher concentrations, destroying the capsid with oxidation. Viruses have no protection against oxidative stress.

The influenza virus has been shown to survive for between 5 hours and 7 days on an outside surface; norovirus can survive on surfaces for approximately 4 hours and can withstand most disinfectants. Ozone gas has been successfully tested against the SARS coronavirus and currently research is ongoing in China at the Institute of Virology in Hubei to establish if it is effective against COVID-19. It has also been tested again polio virus, rotavirus, parvovirus and Hepatitis A and B.[4]

Action Plan

Plug in ozone machines: Ozone generators are able to make ozone from normal air and are used to disinfect and freshen rooms. These can be bought inexpensively off the internet and used to neutralise viral spread in the home. If you have a socket inside a cupboard, for example, plug in a small ozone machine and place any coats and shoes, parcels and packages or supermarket foods and deliveries inside. After a few hours all germs should be destroyed.

Ozonated olive oil is an inexpensive remedy that has been used to help heal a myriad of health problems including eczema, sores and skin lesions, acne, fungal infections and herpes. Ozone is bubbled through the olive oil for several days, until it solidifies into a Vaseline type consistency salve, which can be stored for months in your fridge without losing any of its healing properties. This seems to be the only natural way to stabilise the ozone, without adding chemicals or preservatives.

Invest in a Diffuser: Experiment with a few drops (3-5 drops) of anti-viral essential oils (see p.68 for a comprehensive list) in a diffuser to keep your rooms purified. Add a few drops to a carrier oil such as coconut or olive oil and rub into your skin before you venture out to the supermarket; or dab onto a tissue and sniff up your nose to keep your nasal passages and lungs clear.

Heat as an Anti-viral

Most viruses thrive in the cold, which is why winter is the most dangerous time for catching a cold or falling prey to viral infection. When the warmer seasons arrive, the number of infections may decrease. MERS, which is also a coronavirus, was slowed in its transmission as the environment became warmer and more humid.[5]

A temperature of 70-120 C (165-250F) will destroy most bacteria and some viruses, though not all. Many germs are inactivated by heat – boiling water kills most germs, as does cooking at a higher temperature. Canned food similarly is heat treated to prevent the multiplication of germs over the course of its shelf life. The World Health Organisation states that coronaviruses in general, which includes MERS, SARS and the common cold, can be destroyed at around 70˚C.[6]

Action Plan

Gargling: Try and drink water throughout the day to keep your throat and mouth moist. If a virus enters your mouth, either through touching something or breathing it in from the air, it can enter your windpipe and get into your lungs, which are susceptible to viral attack. Regularly drinking something warm every half an hour or so keeps your mouth clear and will wash any microbes into your stomach where the acid will destroy the majority of them. Gargling with salt in warm water, or lemon or apple cider vinegar in warm water, will act as a preventative.

If you develop any signs of a sore throat attack it immediately – viruses enter the system via the throat and remain there for 3 or 4 days before passing into the lungs.

Inhalation: Many plant- based oils help fight infection and colds and inhaling them, with your head covered with a cloth over a bowl of scented steaming water, is an effective way of freeing up breathing and easing respiratory conditions. Pour a few drops of cinnamon oil, oregano oil and eucalyptus oil onto a wad of cotton wool and inhale deeply. The Australian aborigines have been using the technique successfully for virally triggered respiratory illness for centuries.

Sauna: A normal sauna heats from the outside in; a far-infra red sauna from the inside out. Either way, set the heat control dial high and there is a good possibility of destroying some viruses before they can take a hold.

Saunas, used therapeutically, can recreate the internal effects of a fever, without any of the discomfort. At 102°F (39°C) cancer cells are said to die; at 104°F (40°C) the polio virus has been shown to get stopped in its tracks and the pneumonia bacterium is wiped out at 106°F (41.1°C). In a 1959-review of studies on the effects of heat treatments, Mayo Clinic researcher Dr Wakim and colleagues found that the number of white blood cells in the blood increased by an average of 58% during artificially induced fever.[7]

Steam: A steam in your local gym is another form of heat therapy, though the plus points of the therapy may be outweighed by the risk of contagion by other users. The temperature inside a steam room is usually between 110-114°F (43-45.5°C) with a humidity level of 100%. Benefits include a lowering of blood pressure levels and improved circulation, possibly due to a release of 'feel good' endorphins due to the heat. Regular use has been shown to kill off cold and flu viruses and ease sore throats and lung congestion. White blood cell production increases.[8]

Swop your usual cup of something hot for an anti-viral tea: Herbal teas are an effective way to protect against viruses. Steep a tablespoon of the herb of your choice in hot water for 5-10 minutes and then drink. Both Thyme and Oregano tea reduce levels of candida and mould in the intestines which will be preventing your 'good' gut bacteria functioning optimally. Try mixing the two together with lemon juice and a drop of manuka honey.

Or make a stronger version – a herbal infusion. This draws out the enzymes, minerals, vitamins and other nutrients into the drink. Soak 4 tablespoons of antiviral herbs in boiling water, leave overnight and then drink it hot or cold. The longer the herbs are steeped, the stronger the flavour. Don't drink more than a single cup of this in a 24-hour period.

Echinacea tea: In tests echinacea was effective against all strains of human and avian influenza viruses as well as herpes simplex virus, the common cold and several respiratory viruses, reducing virally triggered inflammation in the tissues.[9]

Olive leaf tea is a scientifically proven anti-viral and immune system booster.[10]

Cats Claw tea is anti-inflammatory and has been show to effectively combat herpes and HIV. It is also said to work against the Epstein-Barr virus. Combine eight ounces of water with a tablespoon of the herb and soak. Drink in the evening. If you buy the tincture, make sure it is not alcohol based which reduces the efficacy of the herb.[11]

Green tea has been shown to inhibit HIV, herpes simplex and the Hepatitis B virus. It contains catechins which are flavonoids that stop the virus replicating.

Pau d'Arco tea contains quinoids, which damage the DNA and RNA of viral proteins, preventing them from breaking through the cell walls of their intended host and reproducing.[12]

CHAPTER TEN

MAKE YOUR OWN ANTI-VIRAL HOME SOLUTIONS

Natural health solutions work every bit as effectively around the house as many of the supermarket options. They can also help soothe sore throats, stomach upsets, and alleviate many of the symptoms of pneumonia, fever, cough and breathing difficulties. Learn to make your own in times when you simply don't feel up to going to the shops.

Clean Up the Bugs

What happens when the supermarkets run out of cleaning products? Make your own from baking soda, lemon and vinegar. Bicarbonate of soda is the UK and Australia's equivalent of the American name for baking soda. Both are the same thing. Vinegar contains acetic acid which kills viruses by chemically changing the proteins and fats inside them and destroying their cellular structure.[1] Disinfect all cans and bottles before you drink from them.

Viruses can survive on surfaces for hours and even days. Tests on COVID-19 found it remained 'virulent' on surfaces from up to 24 hours on cardboard to two or three days on plastic and stainless steel[2]. Poisoning them with bleach (4 teaspoons per litre) is toxic for most germs, distorting their molecules as you sterilize the surfaces. Also note that bleach and bleach alternatives are intended to disinfect surfaces, and should not be used on the skin, and that bleach should never be combined with ammonia or ammonia-based cleaners[3].

If you prefer a more natural solution, vinegar has disinfectant properties, although it is not effective against the coronavirus that causes COVID-19. A 10% malt vinegar solution has, however, been shown to de-activate the influenza virus.[4]

Anti-viral Surface Cleaner
Ingredients

- White distilled vinegar

- Water

- Lemon

- Eucalyptus, rosemary and cinnamon essential oils

Mix 50:50 distilled white vinegar and water in a spray bottle, with 3.5 tablespoons of lemon and 20 drops of a combination of cinnamon, eucalyptus and rosemary essential oils for your surfaces.

Combine vinegar and bicarbonate of soda, and you get a chemical re-action that makes cleaning your toilet relatively fun! Spray the inside of your toilet bowl with distilled white vinegar until it's completely wet. Sprinkle some bicarbonate of soda onto the wet surface, and stand back and watch it fizz. Wait five minutes, then scrub the toilet bowl thoroughly with a toilet brush.

Anti-viral hand sanitiser

Ingredients

- Aloe vera gel

- Tea tree oil

- Vitamin E oil

- Surgical spirit

- Distilled water

- Essential oils of your choice (see p.68)

First find a bottle – glass, if possible, because some essential oils are strong and can degrade plastic. A darker colour protects the life and strength of the oils.

Your local health food store will stock aloe vera gel and tea tree oil and you can buy distilled water and surgical spirit at your nearest pharmacy (also called rubbing alcohol or Isopropyl alcohol). You will need a bottle of 60-95% alcohol. Vodka and gin won't work effectively enough!

Several studies have found that adding alcohol kills more viruses and in greater numbers than a sanitiser with a lower alcohol concentration, or no alcohol at all.

Take a mixing bowl and add between 5-10 drops of the oils of your choice to the aloe vera gel. A few additional drops of vitamin E oil will soften the skin of your hands. Pour it all into your bottle and shake thoroughly. Top up with alcohol (at least 60% alcohol content to enable penetration of the viruses protective coating) and then your distilled water and shake again. A balanced ratio is 60% alcohol: 20% distilled water: 20% aloe vera gel.

> **Top Tip:** Commercial hand sanitisers leave a light film on your hands, and will not protect you from viruses indefinitely. They also disrupt your hand microbiome.[5] Only use a maximum of 5 times before washing thoroughly with soap and water.

Anti-viral room spray

Coronavirus is an airborne virus. It travels through the air, and when you breathe it in it takes hold inside your body. Logically, therefore, enveloping it with potent antivirals in that same space should stop it in its tracks before it has a chance to gain a foothold.

There are three major entry points for it to penetrate your defences - via your nose and mouth and your eyes. Cover these bases and your odds of catching it before it can do extensive harm may well increase.

Stock up with the anti-viral essential oils of your choice (see p.68) and mix them together in combination for a potent and delicious smelling protective defence. Spray into the air around you and squirt into the back of your throat and even up your nose. (Never, however, spray neat essentials oils anywhere near your eyes or you could cause serious damage)

Ingredients

*   Distilled water

*   Essential oils

*   Salt

*   Witch hazel

It's very simple. First find a small glass spray bottle. Buy a bottle of distilled water from the pharmacy, choose your essential oils and you are good to go. 6 oz water with 20-25 drops of different oils should both smell sweet and offer some degree of protection.

If you are going to be using and topping up the spray frequently, you don't need a preservative such as vodka or witch hazel, but as oil and water always struggle to mix, make sure you shake your bottle thoroughly before squirting. As an alternative you can add a teaspoon of salt, which helps with a smoother emulsification.

Drop in your chosen oils, add the teaspoon of salt and shake well, adding the water gradually last of all.

How to make your own Fruit and Vegetable Cleaning Solution

Ingredients

- White distilled vinegar

- Water

Make a 50/50 water/vinegar solution and rinse fruit and vegetables thoroughly. In one test using a vinegar wash was found to reduce the numbers of viruses on strawberries by 95%.[6]

Soap works well too, breaking through the viral membranes and destroying them. Just make sure you rinse extremely well before eating.

> **Top Tip:** Wash your clothes at a temperature of 60° or higher, which will destroy most viruses.

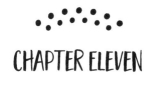

CHAPTER ELEVEN

EMOTIONS AND IMMUNITY

Anti-viral Emotional Defence

The Power of Positive Thought

Feeling depressed and anxious at the thought of being cut off from your family and friends and facing the oncoming weeks full of fear and dread? What can you do to fill the endless hours while you wait for the virus to pass? Thinking positively can be very hard when you are feeling overwhelmed and stressed. But there are very good reasons why it is important to try. Your state of mind – and spirit – are closely linked to the strength of your immunity. As the developmental biologist, Bruce Lipton, explains in his remarkable book, *The Biology of Belief*, specific strong feelings like grief, anger, revenge, fear or depression trigger strong associated chemicals, such as cortisol and adrenaline, which, if released into your bloodstream daily over a long period of time, can have a detrimental impact on your brain. But changing your way of thinking can help you to take back control of your mental health and your brain function. Choosing to behave and think in ways that flood your body with positive feelings (gratitude, joy, peace and love) on a daily basis has a powerful physiological impact on the wellbeing of your body (and brain) because of the chemicals associated with those feelings.

Action Plan

Time	Mon	Tue	Wed	Thur	Fri	Sat	Sun

Design a Day to Day Timetable

Set up a structure for passing your day, and then stick to it. Fill in each hour with something constructive to do – or not to do – and your mind will relax because it knows and understands its direction. Leaving it all up in the air is more likely to trigger thoughts and feelings that lead you in a negative direction. And when you finally emerge from your viral 'forced holiday' you may find you have a collection of new positive habits and daily practices that will continue to improve your mood for years to come.

Filling the Days

- **Meditate** - Boost your mood and reduce stress. (see p.114)

- **Take your anti-viral supplements** (see p.62)

- **Read a book** – learn something new

- **Cooking** – take the time to prepare meals with care. Experiment with new recipes – however restricted your foodstuff.

- **Exercise at home** - It's good for your body and your mind

- **Go for a walk** - Any time spent outdoors makes you happier

- **Sign up for a blog** – obviously I am going to be recommending my own health blog – reboothealth. co.uk. Other favourites include thejproject.co.uk and mummywasasecretdrinker.blogspot.com. I love real peoples stories about overcoming adversity.

- **Listen to your favourite music** – it can lower your stress levels as well as reduce the risk of heart failure.[1]

- **Choose a new hobby** - Ever thought of Origami? Or on-line chess?

- **Talk to family and friends** – either on the phone or zoom or FaceTime them.

continued...

Top Tip: Keep connected: Download the Houseparty app which allows you to talk to, and see, a group of different friends all at the same time. Schedule a daily catch up.

- **Email time** – reconnect with friends you haven't been in touch with for years

- **Play computer games** – whether it's the addictive Candy Crush, Solitaire or the more constructive BrainHQ app which gives you exercises to stimulate your memory and sharpen up your brain

- **Sort your cupboards** – fill up a few bin bags with the unwanted items that have sat there for ages. Learn how to use eBay to sell anything you haven't used for years.

- **House cleaning time** – don't forget light switches, toilet flushes and door handles!

- **Garden** if you have access to an outside space. And if you don't, offer to garden in someone else's!

- **Time for Gratitude** – write a diary and list the top 5 things you have been grateful for that day. They can be as simple as the joyous thought of a newly blossomed flower.

- **Think** – about your job, your relationships, your future. Take the time.

continued...

> - **Book in some home cinema time** - sign up for Netflix, AppleTV and circulate any good films to your nearest and dearest - save them the stress of searching through the thousands of available choices.

Get technology savvy

Whatever your age and technological stage, this can be an opportunity for learning. You have been given the unexpected gift of time, and once you are feeling strong enough, can take it and use it for your future benefit. If you have never had an iphone or ipad – and your time at home seems likely to be long, then please get one, and learn how to use it.

Oddly, in these times of social media addiction, it may set you free. It will keep you in touch with your friends and relatives – seeing their faces as well as hearing their voices – and gives you access to a world of information that may have been previously unknown.

You can play games on it – watch YouTube videos and gain access to the world of Kindle books – thousands upon thousands of titles without having to step outside of your front door. Hours of fascination – and education. Most of it for free. Never really learnt to cook? This could be the time. Always wanted to speak a foreign language? Now's your opportunity. Sign up for an online course that upgrades your current level of technology skills. Learn how to use Instagram and Facebook; what Mailchimp does or Squarespace. It's never too late to become a blogger – if you are at home long enough, why not write a book? There are plenty of people explaining exactly how to go about it!

Isolation

Careful here. There is consistent research that links social isolation and loneliness to cardiovascular and mental health problems. It's easy enough to get depressed or anxious at the feeling of being trapped in a far smaller space than normal. Not being able to get out to pass the time of day with friends and neighbours can seem a huge loss to quality of life.[2]

And being confined in a small space with relatives you struggle to get on with can be difficult. Enforced contact with even our nearest and dearest can cause tempers to fray and trigger difficult emotions.

What is going on in your mind and emotions unquestionably affects the body. Boosting your natural immunity level is the number one way to fend off viral infection yet the immune system is quantifiably affected by conflict or trauma. Grief, loneliness, simmering resentment, boredom, anger, jealousy and hatred will all lower your defence mechanisms.

Take control of your mind and use the enforced time to resolve any outstanding issues. Perhaps use it to design the life you always wanted but never had time to focus on creating. Every grey cloud is said to have a silver lining.

Perhaps this is it? A gift not a prison sentence? Change your mind and the science says your immunity will strengthen.

Strategies for working from home

It sounds great when you are first told you need to work from home. No more commuting, rushing after work to do the supermarket run, missing the parcel delivery or being late to collect your children from school. But after a short-time many people report feelings of stress; they miss their co-workers and the buzz of office everyday life. Be careful of your mental health; eat properly and exercise regularly to ensure you don't slowly slip into anxiety and depression.

Action Plan

Find a dedicated working area: Don't move from room to room or from kitchen table to sitting room sofa. Find your spot and stick to it, so your mind knows it's now in 'office mode'. If you dress up in your usual work clothes you may find you work more efficiently too. And stick to your normal working routine: work the hours you always do.

Limit the amount of time you spend listening to the news or reading the papers: Restrict yourself to half an hour a day – once a day - and you will limit the panic and fear that the media can spread so rapidly.

Eat Properly: It's all too easy, if you are confined to your house, to reward yourself with mini breaks – reaching for a biscuit, grabbing another cup of coffee – and your diet can deteriorate. Make sure you have healthy, immune boosting food easily to hand, and restrict the snacks. The weight can pile on – and we've all heard that irritating adage that's been proven far too true a myriad of times - 'a minute on the lips, a lifetime on the hips'. Take action now and that won't be you!

Set your body, set your mind, positively: Do what you've always done on a normal working day – even when you are working from home. Wash your hair, put on your make-up, and don't spend the day in your pyjamas. Repeating the actions of your usual routine will boost your mind and stop you from falling into sloppy habits.

Ban social media: Resist the temptation to be always checking FaceBook and Instagram. Check in in your lunchbreak or after working hours.

Keep work time separate from family time: Set your work boundaries with others in your house. No popping in for a chat while you are in work mode, walking the dog, playing with children or being asked to mend that long broken cupboard door.

Keep connected to your colleagues: use Zoom, FaceTime or Skype and schedule regular one on one video talks and group conferences. Being isolated can be lonely and lead to feelings of depression. Draw up a timetable to keep you on track.

Make the time for regular breaks outdoors: Fresh air and exercise will keep your body fitter and your mind focused.

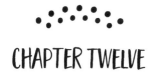

CHAPTER TWELVE

STRESS RELIEF: UNLOAD YOUR BURDEN

Stress is the number one cause of mental exhaustion. It consumes energy voraciously and lowers immunity. Everyday worries – about work or financial difficulties, traffic jams, personal relationships or even the everyday news on the radio and TV – trigger a build-up of stress. Eventually, if the stress is not dealt with, you find yourself temporarily unable to think or function; it's rather like trying to drive in the fast lane of a motorway with the handbrake on. When you are stressed you release large quantities of cortisol, which suppresses the immune system, reducing your natural defences against illness and viruses.

Stress also creates acidity in your physical body, another reason, whilst under viral attack, to release and reduce it as fast as possible.

First, establish your current stress levels
The Energy Scan

High levels of stress quickly deplete energy levels, so take a moment to tune in and check how stressed you are. Sit quietly somewhere and really listen to how your body is feeling.

Imagine that there is a battery inside you – a store of energy – powering your body and marked with the numbers 1–10 at regular intervals from bottom to top.

1.   On that 1–10 scale, how full is your battery?

2.   Write down the number that instantly springs into your mind, along with the date.

3.   You can refer back to it in a few weeks' time when you've had a chance to introduce some of the rebalancing suggestions in this book. Then re-test again and compare the results.

Identify Your Stresses – Past and Present
Just how stressed are you right now?

Have you ever taken the time to sit down and examine the things in your life that cause you pain or that you struggle to cope with? If the answer is no, then this may well be the perfect opportunity for dealing with those issues – and there are a number of effective therapies that you can do in the comfort of your own home, which will happily, and productively, pass the oncoming days.

Action Plan
Keep a Stress Diary

Write down the things that stress you daily – as they happen. It is rare to have a day without having something to record, and seeing it written in black and white on the page, and watching the list build over a period of a week may just surprise you. At the very least it will incentivise you to take steps to reduce your load.

Have a look at the inventory of life stresses chart below[1]. How many of these events have happened to you in the last 12 months? Answering the questions and adding up your score will give you a fairly accurate picture of the stress you are under now.

Life event	Mean value
Death of a spouse/partner	100
Divorce	73
Separation from spouse/partner	65
Detention in jail or other institution	63
Death of a close family member	63
Major personal injury or illness	53
Marriage	50
Being fired from work	47
Reconciliation with spouse/partner	45
Retirement from work	45
Major change in the health or behaviour of family member	44
Pregnancy	40
Sexual difficulties	39
Gaining new family member (through birth, adoption, or older adult moving in)	39
Major business readjustment	39

Major change in financial position (either a lot better off or worse off)	38
Death of a close friend	37
Changing to a different line of work	36
Major change in number of arguments with spouse (either a lot more or a lot less than usual, regarding, for example, childrearing, personal habits etc.)	35
Taking on a mortgage or loan (for home or business)	31
Foreclosure on a mortgage or loan (for home or business)	30
Major change in responsibilities at work (either promotion or demotion)	29
Son or daughter leaving home (for example, for college, marriage, or employment)	29
Difficulties with your partner's family	29
Outstanding personal achievement	28
Spouse/partner beginning or stopping work outside the home	26
Beginning or ceasing formal schooling	26
Major change in living conditions (moving home, deterioration of neighbourhood or home)	25
Major revision to personal habits (e.g. quitting smoking/alcohol, changes to dress, manners or associations)	24
Troubles with your boss	23
Major changes to working hours or conditions	20
Changes in residence	20
Changing schools	20
Major change in usual type and/or amount of recreational activity	19
Major change in church activity (more or less than usual)	19
Major change in social activities (clubs, movies, visiting friends etc.)	18
Taking out a loan for a car, household furniture/ appliances	17

Major change in sleeping habits (much more or much less than usual)	16
Major change in number of family get-togethers	15
Major change in eating habits (a lot more or less than usual, or very different mealtimes or surroundings)	15
Vacation	13
Major holiday	12
Minor violations (speeding or parking fines, disturbing the peace etc.)	11

Now add up your results

150 points or fewer shows a relatively low amount of life change and a low susceptibility to stress-induced health breakdown.

150 to 300 points indicates a 50 per cent chance of health breakdown in the next two years.

300 points or more indicates an 80 per cent chance of health breakdown in the next two years.

Exercise 1: Create a de-stress route map

What would make your life more the one you want it to be, and minimise the stress you are under? The stresses of everyday life can seem to make you rush from pillar to post, and weeks, months and even years, pass in a flash. You may be 'surviving', but it can feel as if life is running you; you are not creating its content and direction.

Life rarely gives you the time to consciously consider what would give you the most satisfaction in the long term.

Take that time now. Accept the time you now have to spend indoors as an unexpected gift from any virus not a burden. Simply change your mind and the way you see the situation. Taking back control of your thoughts is vital in any attempt to boost your immune system and strengthen it against viral attack.

Sit quietly and alone and take your time to consider what would really make your heart sing – might it be moving to a new home, travelling, finding a partner, changing job or getting a pet? Take as long as you need, let your mind pop the answers into your head.

Write down your answers, in as much detail as possible. You may be surprised at what arises when you really listen to yourself.

The mind works on instructions, so once you are clear on where you want to go, and what changes are needed to make it happen, set this as a clear intention for your future, then repeat it to yourself constantly. Imagine the change in the present – for example the new buyers (of the flat you haven't been able to sell for months, because the message you are sending to your mind daily is 'the flat's not selling') are asking which pieces of furniture they can buy.

The mind does exactly what it is told, always. It can't distinguish between reality and imagined reality. It merely follows the instructions it is given and does its best to deliver that instruction. Chaotic thoughts and negative messaging will deliver chaotic and negative results to your door. Similarly, a mental image of your new life will deliver a concrete plan to you.

Exercise 2: Write out your past stresses

While identifying your present difficulties is a good wake-up call, what about more deeply buried stresses and traumas in your past?

We all deal with difficult experiences in different ways and what seems small and bearable to one person may feel like the end of the world to another. If, in the present, you can still remember, see and feel what happened many years earlier, then that event is still 'live' in your non-conscious mind.

To move past stresses out of your brain, try the next exercise.

Get a notebook, then sit still (or even lie down) for a few minutes in a quiet room. Shut your eyes and ask your mind to send you images of anything that needs resolving; let memories and pictures flood your mind. People, places and things that you haven't thought of for years will come into your head, some of them seemingly insignificant, and some with unexpected clarity.

Write everything down – just use short headings that you can use to jog your memory later. It may be anything, from when you fell off the sofa as a baby, your first difficult day at secondary school, failing an exam, to ending your first relationship, losing your job, your dog dying, being left by a partner, or the death of a parent. The pressures of everyday life are endless and varied.

The list, and its length, will be different for everyone. Some people will focus on events from years ago, and others on more recent happenings. If you have been under a lot of stress recently, your recall for long-past events will be slower, but surprising connections will still appear. What is important is that you keep writing until no more pictures and memories come into your head; it doesn't matter how long that list becomes.

Each memory carries a portion of all the stress your system is experiencing and adds to your sense of psychological burden. Bringing them into your conscious mind is the first step on the path to realising their past significance, and then releasing their current intrusive hold over you. Some will take more effort to re-organise than others. For the experiences and memories that affect you most deeply, long-term talking therapy may be required, but others can be worked through with simple self-directed exercises at home. It doesn't require much time. Even dealing with one event a day over a period of 30 days will reduce your stress burden considerably.

How to reduce stress

- **Try Tapping**

Emotional Freedom Technique, or EFT, combines positive affirmations with the tapping of acupressure points, and is a simple and effective way to release negative thoughts and emotions and deeply held emotional and physical traumas. It works seamlessly alongside any medical treatments you are receiving from your GP or surgeon and has no side effects of any kind.

The theory is that stress and trauma can prevent the body's energy from flowing smoothly and build up blockages that eventually manifest as physical problems, lowering your immunity at the same time. Gentle tapping on specific acupressure points, however, vibrates through the meridians, clearing those blockages and bringing the body back to balance, releasing difficult thoughts and feelings at the same time.

It is an easy healing method to learn yourself as the same eight points are tapped in the same sequence, no matter what the illness or problem is. You can work in the privacy of your own home and it can take as little as a single session to resolve even the most traumatic issue. 'Step-by-Step Tapping' by Emma Roberts and Sue Beer is a helpful guide.

- **Mental Health Healing Apps**

You can now access help for mental health issues simply at the touch of a button on your phone. Want to have your symptoms diagnosed and assessed? Or just talk to an expert? A problem shared very often makes all the difference.

You need never feel alone in your troubles.

1. **Talkspace:** This is a counselling and therapy app that offers a free initial consultation with a specialist from their database of over 1,000 qualified therapists skilled in treating depression, anxiety, stress, phobias, PTSD and domestic violence. When you find the right therapist for you there is the option to become a member and discuss your issues in a private online chat room, at less than 80% of the cost of conventional therapy sessions.

2. **What's Up?** This free app uses CBT techniques (Cognitive Behavioural Therapy) alongside ACT (Acceptance Commitment Therapy) to help you deal with anger, stress, depression and anxiety. Find out what the 12 most common negative thinking patterns are and learn how to overcome them. Keep a diary of your emotions daily and track any changes.

3. **Anxiety Relief Hypnosis:** Hypnosis de-stresses your mind and reduces anxiety and difficult thoughts and feelings. This free app offers an audio session with a registered hypnotherapist, alongside relaxing music and sounds from nature to lower your stress levels. It is said to re-set your reactions and lessen anxiety levels within the space of 1-3 weeks.

4. **SuperBetter** is a game app that helps you to remain strong and optimistic even when life throws you lemons. A study by the University of Pennsylvania found that after participants played it regularly for a month, their anxiety levels decreased and their overall mood improved along with their belief in their ability to succeed in life. The app

claims to help you 'adopt new hab
strengthen relationships, complet
and fulfill life-long dreams'. Alon
cope with chronic illness and rec
and anxiety. Who could ask for mc

Emo

5. **Pacifica:** an app that aims to reduce anxiety, stress and depression by setting you challenges involving audio lessons and targeted activities. It uses meditation, mindfulness and CBT, alongside other relaxation methods and tracks your mood daily. It offers a toolbox to break the mental habits that don't serve you and also offers access to a community of like-minded people to help and support you to break free from overwhelming stress.

6. **7cups:** an online emotional support service that gives you someone to talk to for free. Their database contains over 160,000 trained listeners and licensed therapists experienced in stress and anxiety to whom you can speak anonymously in total confidence. You can search for a topic you need help with - bullying, eating disorders, panic attacks, relationship difficulties - and if you choose, then continue with the same advisor, one on one, for longer term counselling.

...ional healing with Bach flower remedies

...scovered by Dr Edward Bach in the early 20th century, these 38 remedies can help you to release difficult to deal with mind states and relieve specific emotions. Scroll through the list and see if any of the emotions relate to you. Grade yourself for the intensity of the feeling – with 10 being an extreme overload, and 0 nothing at all – and write it down so that you can refer back and repeat the test in a couple of weeks.

They are available either online or in most natural health stores. Add a few drops of your chosen remedy to a 30ml bottle of water and take four drops four times a day. There is even a Rescue remedy for emergency stress relief which contains a combination of five essences.[2]

Agrimony for mental torture behind a cheerful face
Aspen for fear of unknown things
Beech for intolerance
Centaury for the inability to say 'no'
Cerato for lack of trust in one's own decisions
Cherry Plum for fear of the mind giving way
Chestnut Bud for failure to learn from mistakes
Chicory for selfish, possessive love
Clematis for dreaming of the future without working in the present
Crab Apple for the cleansing remedy, also for self-hatred
Elm for overwhelmed by responsibility
Gentian for discouragement after a setback
Gorse for hopelessness and despair

Heather for self-centredness and self-concern

Holly for hatred, envy and jealousy

Honeysuckle for living in the past

Hornbeam for tiredness at the thought of doing something

Impatiens for impatience

Larch for lack of confidence

Mimulus for fear of known things

Mustard for deep gloom for no reason

Oak for the plodder who keeps going past the point of exhaustion

Olive for exhaustion following mental or physical effort

Pine for guilt

Red chestnut for over-concern for the welfare of loved ones

Rock rose for terror and fright

Rock water for self-denial, rigidity and self-repression

Scleranthus for inability to choose between alternatives

Star of Bethlehem for shock

Sweet chestnut for extreme mental anguish, when everything has been tried and there is no light left

Vervain for over-enthusiasm

Vine for dominance and inflexibility

Walnut for protection from change and unwanted influences

Water violet for quiet self-reliance leading to isolation

White chestnut for unwanted thoughts and mental arguments

Wild oat for uncertainty over one's direction in life

Wild rose for drifting, resignation, apathy

Willow for self-pity and resentment

Meditate

Meditation is highly recommended if you are one of the one in four people who suffers from mental ill health, including anxiety or depression. You may already be aware of Headspace, with its vast selection of mindfulness and meditation sessions or Calm, which was Apple's app of the year of 2017 and focuses on relaxation, sleep, breathing and meditation. Both of them offer an extensive selection of tools to calm your mind and release stress.

In a 2013 study[3], 93 people who had been diagnosed with generalised anxiety disorder were assigned to a mindfulness group for eight weeks, whilst another group received stress management advice.4 Those who did the mindfulness programme experienced a significantly greater reduction in their symptoms. Similarly, research from the University of Oxford found that a mindfulness intervention was more effective at helping prevent a recurrence of depressive episodes than antidepressant medication.

How to meditate

Whether this is your first-time meditating, or you've explored it before, the key thing to remember is that while the benefits are instant, they are also incremental. Committing to regular meditation will deliver brain-changing benefits over time with practice (and patience). Don't expect it to be easy. It's quite normal to find that as soon as you try to still your mind, your brain is overrun by a whole load of unwanted and unwelcome thoughts. This is

NOT a sign that you are 'bad' at meditation, or that it won't work for you. The key is to simply notice your distracting thoughts and move on, trying as far as you can to resist letting them lead you away from your breath, or your point of focus.

Morning meditation

This is a mindfulness meditation designed to energise you and help you improve your ability to focus and concentrate. It is a great way to counteract an anxious, over-busy brain. Aim to practise this for ten minutes as soon as possible after waking.

1. Sit with a relaxed, upright spine and close your eyes.

2. Begin to focus on your breath, draw the air deep down to the very bottom of your lungs. Notice the sensation of air flowing into your nostrils for a count of four, pause for a moment at the top of the breath.

3. Exhale for a count of four. Repeat.

4. Repeat the in and out breaths as above for 10 minutes, focusing on them at all times. Whenever thoughts intrude, draw your attention back to your breath.

Practise Yoga Nidra daily

This is a meditation technique where you consciously relax each part of your body, one area at a time. This refocuses your brain, and relaxes your body, releasing tension and allowing you, within a short period of time, to slip gently back into sleep. Start by relaxing all the muscles in your face and head, including your tongue, jaw, and eyes. Drop your shoulders as low as they'll go. Then relax your arms, first on one side, and then the other. Move your attention next to your chest, and relax every part of it. Then relax your legs, releasing any muscle tension in your calves and thighs. Once all stress has vanished physically, relax your mind as well. Find your special tranquil place - imagine yourself rocking gently in a rowing boat, on a calm lake under a blue sky, or lying on a white beach next to a turquoise sea.

Dr Munshi's Breathing Exercise

This is the technique developed by a doctor and nurses at Queens Hospital in Romford to help patients with respiratory problems fight off the coronavirus infection and strengthen their lungs. It is a rapid way of getting additional air into the lungs.

How to do it:

1. Take five deep breaths in, holding in between each for five seconds before breathing out.

2. On the sixth breath, as you exhale, cough deeply (covering your mouth, into your hands or shirt)

3. Repeat again for a second round

4. Then lie on your front for 10 mins, with pillow under your front, taking deep but shorter breaths.

Stress reducing technology

Touchpoints

Research shows that a pair of small rectangular pulsing 'Touchpoints' can release approximately 70% of stress from your brain in a matter of minutes, just by holding them in the palm of your hands - or wearing them on your wrists.

They are extremely simple to use. They use bi-lateral alternating stimulation technology (BLAST) to restore calm in your brain and boost rational thinking. In 'normal' speak what they do is buzz and vibrate - at a different rate and timing in each hand, over-riding the brain's habitual patterns and in the process releasing any stress build up.[4]

Anti-anxiety AcuPips

These are tiny 'ear seeds' - acupressure tools that help you bring the benefits of acupuncture to your own home. Simply apply to 3 specific points on your ear and replace every three days to relieve your anxiety levels. Backed with sticky clear tape, they are hardly noticeable as they work to calm your nervous system. Research shows that they may stimulate activity in the brain, reducing stress immediately. They were used successfully after 9/11, Hurricane Katrina and the California wildfires to help deal with trauma.[5]

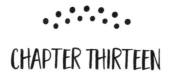

CHAPTER THIRTEEN

CORONAVIRUS – A GLOBAL PANDEMIC

There are hundreds of coronaviruses in existence, but only seven to-date are thought to have 'jumped' across from animals to infect humans. These include SARS (Severe acute respiratory syndrome) and MERS (Middle East respiratory syndrome). The World Health Organisation has declared the new coronavirus COVID-19 outbreak a pandemic - a global outbreak of a disease. To-date, approximately 81% of people who are infected have mild cases, however for others the disease can be fatal.[1]

COVID-19 Facts And Figures

COVID-19 is an airborne virus. It travels through the air, and you breathe it in. It has an incubation period of around 14 days.[2] Symptoms are usually initially mild and similar to those of a normal cold including fevers, coughs and difficulty breathing. Many infected people show no symptoms at all but in severe cases the disease can develop into serious pneumonia-like disease.

Few of us currently have immunity against this newly mutated superbug and between countries, fatality rates vary significantly.[3] Those who are thought to be most susceptible are people suffering from lung and heart disease. The frail elderly with stressed immune systems caused by chronic diseases such as diabetes, asthma, respiratory diseases and cardiovascular issues are the most at risk. Men are more susceptible to infection than women; children under the age of 9 seem rarely affected.

If the infection goes on multiplying at the rate it is currently, it's probably best, if you are feeling unwell and are concerned you may have it, not to go to the hospital, or to a clinic, where you may well either pass the virus on to others, or pick it up from someone similarly worried. Instead, stay at home, and, if you are in the UK, call 111. They will, apparently, send medical help to you directly.

The R0 number

There is a mathematical term that indicates how contagious an infectious disease is likely to be – the R0 (pronounced R nought) number. R0 tells you the average number of people that will catch that disease from a single contagious person. It applies to large groups of people who haven't been vaccinated and were previously free of contagion, and is particularly valuable looking at countries exposed to an entirely new virus where there is no way to control the disease.

The higher the number the longer the infection period is likely to be. The 1918 outbreak of the Spanish Flu (the swine flu H1N1 virus) had an R0 value estimated at between 1.4 and 2.8. The more recent swine flu outbreak in 2009 had a R0 value of 1.4 -1.6.[4]

The measles virus has an R0 number of 18; mumps has one of 10, SARS 4, HIV 4, Ebola 2 and Hepatitis C an R0 of 2. The flu virus has an R0 of 1.3, and the virus SARS-CoV-2, the virus that causes the disease COVID-19, is estimated at about 2.2, meaning a single infected person on average will infect about 2.2 others.

Animal contagion

The COVID-19 virus shares about 90% of its genetic material with coronaviruses that infect bats, which suggests that the virus originated in bats and later moved on to humans probably via another animal. SARS was tracked from bats to civets and then on to infect humans. MERS infected camels before spreading to humans.

Approximately 50% of us own a pet but at present there is no evidence that pets can be a source of COVID-19. Cats and dogs develop their own versions of coronavirus (CCV) and (FIP) but these cannot be transmitted to humans.[5] On the flip side, however, cases have been reported of owners transmitting the disease to their pets.

COVID-19 Symptoms

You may not show signs of symptoms for up to two weeks after infection, although signs and symptoms on average develop 5-6 days after infection.[6]

1. Patients develop a new continuous cough and a high temperature.

2. Approximately 1/3 of people will produce sputum.

3. Only around 5% of patients will develop a runny nose, sneezing or sore throat

4. Patients report muscle pain and shortness of breath after about a week.

5. The virus then develops into a nasal fluid that enters the trachea and the lungs, triggering severe inflammation and pneumonia. This lasts approximately 6 more days and is accompanied by a high fever and breathing difficulties.

6. Patients also report a 100% loss of the senses of taste and smell.

According to the World Health Organisation, based on 55,924 cases, percentages of typical signs and symptoms are as follows:

Fever - 87%; Dry Cough - 67.7%; Fatigue - 38.1%; sputum production - 33.4%; shortness of breath - 18.6%; sore throat - 13.9%; headache - 13.6%; myalgia or arthralgia - 14.8%; chills - 11.4%; nausea or vomiting - 5%; nasal congestion - 4.8%; diarrhoea - 3.7%.[7]

Flattening the curve: This is a term used to describe attempts being made by the Government to mitigate the effects of an infectious virus, on both the population and the hospital system that has to cope with any outbreak. It includes limiting the symptoms of the virus before unmanageable numbers of the population become infected; limiting the rate of spread of infection; and speeding up the time it takes to develop a vaccine

Two strategies are thought to slow the spread of the virus:

Social distancing: This means reducing your contact with other people as much as possible: working from home rather than the office, avoiding public places as well as crowded pubs and restaurants, bus and train stations, and if someone in your home develops signs of a cough or a fever, then staying at home for between 7 and 14 days till the contagious period is over.

Self-isolation: This is taking social distancing a step further, cutting yourself off from the rest of the world and staying inside your home for a period that can range from 14 days to several months. If one person in a household starts to display flu like symptoms, for example – such as a persistent cough or a fever of above 37.8˚C (100.4), everyone living there must stay at home for a fortnight. You are allowed to go outside to exercise as long as you keep at a safe distance from other people, but you need to get foods and household essentials delivered, not go to the shops to buy them yourself.

Potential medical solutions

There are currently no vaccines available for COVID-19, though every research laboratory in the world is doing their best to develop one. Any success will take time and this is likely to be 12-18 months away from being released to the general public. Tests are available now, however, that show whether you have already had the infection and have developed anti-bodies to it. Although there are no specific antiviral drugs to treat this form of human coronavirus, a handful of existing pharmaceutical drugs do exist that may slow the progress of the disease and speed up recovery time.

Chloroquine: This is an inexpensive and relatively safe anti-malarial drug that has been studied as a possible anti-viral for many years. Research has suggested that it hinders the ability of viruses to enter human cells. A trial that involved 36 patients showed that 70 percent of those given it recovered from Covid-19 within 6 days. There are signs that it reduces viral load which might mean that even if you do develop symptoms they may be less severe. It also damps down the inflammatory complications of several viral diseases.[8]

Favipiravir: This is a Japanese flu treatment which trials in China have shown reduces recovery time from COVID-19 to four days compared to 11 days in the control group. It is reported to protect against lung damage and also to work better when administered soon after diagnosis rather than later in the disease's progression.[9]

Remdesivir: This anti-viral drug was originally developed to combat Ebola, and is considered to be generally safe with few side effects. It prevents viruses from replicating and infecting new cells. Trials have already started to test it against COVID-19. Earlier research suggests that it was effective against SARS and MERS.[10]

> **Top Tip:** Stock up on paracetamol in case of infection, but do not take ibuprofen which seems to exacerbate symptoms, with people with no underlying health problems going on to develop serious symptoms, including respiratory complications, after using non-steroidal anti-inflammatory drugs (NSAID's) in the early stage of infection.[11]

Complementary therapies for Coronavirus symptoms relief

Homeopathy for COVID-19

Byronia Alba is the standard remedy for pleurisy, and is recommended for the initial symptoms of coronavirus by homeopathic doctor, Dr Manish Bhatia. Bryonia also dries up mucus and fluid.

He recommends Lycopodium for later symptoms, particularly if sufferers go on to develop pneumonia. Doseages vary according to your symptoms, so it is best to consult a homeopath to get it right. Both Ainsworths and Nelson's Homeopathic Pharmacies have onsite experts.

This was written by Dr. Bhatia

'It can be given (only to affected population) once a day, till days become warmer and the epidemic subsides (hopefully). People who are mobile in endemic or epidemic areas should take the medicine daily. People who are in

self quarantine and not having social contact, can take it for 3-5 days and then take it if and when they venture out. If a patient has flu-like symptoms, you can take the same remedy in 6 or 30 potency, 6 hourly. If the vitality is very low, more frequent repetition may be required. Also consider Camphora in such a case.

If a patient develops tightness in chest and shortness of breath, Lycopodium 30CH is likely to help.

The remedy suggestions are based on the available data. Homeopathy needs much deeper individualization, and clinical experience of treating Coronavirus Covid-19 patients with homeopathy may bring up a different group of remedies.

Some recent data from Iran shows that many patients are showing sudden collapse. Dr. Rajan Sakaran as well as Dr. Sunirmal Sarkar have suggested that Camphora 1M be considered as a medicine and prophylactic there. So if Covid-19 patients in your country are showing signs of sudden collapse with respiratory distress, vertigo and cold sweat, you may consider Camphora.

I do not recommend self-medication. You can show this article to your homeopath for a better clinical judgment that he/she will make for you'.[12]

Acupuncture and acupressure

Viral infection may leave you with a weakness in the lungs. Acupuncture can help to strengthen the area, but if you are at home in bed, then acupressure is the next best thing.

Even a couple of minutes twice a day firmly massaging the points on the hand shown below, will make a difference, relieving pain and fever and alleviating breathing issues and respiratory problems.

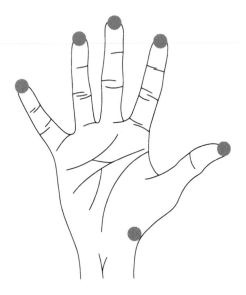

Proning

'Prone positioning' involves placing an intensive care patient onto their stomach for 12 hours, to disperse fluid that has built up in their lungs. The majority of your lung is on your back not on your front, so lying on it compresses and closes off a large area of the smaller airways, leaving you more vulnerable to secondary pneumonia.

Sore Throat

Apple cider vinegar: Sore throats vanish quickly if you gargle with a 50% apple cider vinegar/50% warm water solution. Buy the organic, raw, unprocessed apple cider vinegar, containing what is rather peculiarly called 'the mother', which is the cloudy version with the bits at the bottom. Those bits are strands of proteins, enzymes and good bacteria. Try Braggs apple cider vinegar.

Tea tree oil: Gargle with it to stop a sore throat, or inhale a cloud of tea tree laced steam to clear your sinuses. It's a remarkable all-rounder.

Zinc lozenges: Suck these slowly, keeping them in your throat for 30 minutes at a time. Take 4 or 5 a day.

Propolis: At the first sign of coronavirus symptoms, a sore throat and fever, spray propolis to the back of your throat. In the first 5 days after the virus takes hold, it will multiply in your nasal membranes and propolis has been shown to stimulate anti-viral action in the mucous.[13]

Top Tip: Isotonic HOCL spray is an effective anti-viral to use to disinfect your face, eyes, mouth and hands. HydrOxyChloride (HOCL) is produced naturally by your white blood cells to combat pathogens. Backed by scientific peer-reviewed research, these sprays have been shown to safely destroy bacteria, yeasts, fungus, mould and viruses and yet don't upset the micro flora of your skin. It can also be used as a surface cleaner.[14]

Briotech topical skin spray has been laboratory tested against human coronavirus OC43 and found, after 10 minutes of exposure, to reduce viral infection by 99.9999%. Briotechusa.com.[15]

WiFi

'It has been suggested that recent deaths of younger, apparently healthy, people from COVID-19 may be linked to high levels of WiFi use and/or electro-magnetic fields which are a known cause of decreased melatonin levels. It would seem sensible, therefore, to supplement with melatonin (see p 62) and shield against WiFi wherever possible. Giawellness.com offers a range of patented options backed up by extensive research. Their GIA CellGuard can be used on mobile phones, laptops, iPads, TV's and routers.[16]

Get humming: One of the ways the coronavirus multiplies is by hiding inside your nose, replicating in your sinuses and nasal passages before infecting the rest of your body. One of the symptoms reported is loss of smell, and that may be caused by the virus multiplying there. Somewhat weirdly, humming increases the build-up of nitric oxide in the nose, stopping the virus in its tracks. Humming regularly can apparently both prevent and treat COVID-19.[17]

For those with lung issues a combination of humming and supplementing with vitamin c and melatonin (see p.61 and 62) is thought to halt the triggering of the 'cytokine storm' that creates the severe respiratory conditions and pneumonia associated with COVID-19. For countries that have no access to melatonin, propolis can be used instead.[18]

Headache Relief

One of the distressing symptoms of COVID-19 that seems to linger is an intense headache that normal over-the-counter medicines don't seem to relieve. A simple EFT tapping technique is reported to effectively reduce the pain.

EFT (Emotional Freedom Technique) consists of a series of easy to do at home 'taps' on specific acupuncture meridians, accompanied by specific phrases that instantly release the stress and soothe your head, along with the mental worry that accompanies the physical pain. There are a multitude of YouTube videos that will show you the technique. EFTuniverse.com

'Seven-Step Approach to Migraines using EFT tapping' will talk you through how to do it. Emma Roberts and Sue

Beer's 'Step by Step Tapping' is an excellent book on the topic.

Invest in a pulse oxymeter

These are small devices that clip onto the end of your finger and give a reading on the levels of oxygen in your blood in a matter of seconds. If your baseline reading drops this could be an early warning of infection. COVID-19 pneumonia initially causes 'silent hypoxia', a form of oxygen deprivation, so prompt detection of the problem could lead to earlier treatment, avoiding a later need for ventilation.

Post coronavirus recovery

It seems, from reports from other countries ahead of us in the COVID-19 tables, that recovery is not simply a question of coming through the infection safely, though that for many is an achievement in itself. It now appears that it is possible to catch the virus more than once, and for some people, recovery may take many weeks. Patients speak of aching joints and headaches and non-existent energy levels. One reader described herself as being 'in a black hole', and that was several weeks after she had 'got better'.

The keys that speed recovery

There are, it seems to me, (though none of us have been here before, so this is advice based on logic rather than experience) three principal strategies to follow to speed up recovery.

Address underlying health conditions

The first must be to resolve any underlying health conditions that you suffer from as much as is possible. Alongside upping your exercise levels, a healthy diet and lifestyle can reverse even diabetes and high blood pressure.

Read my book 'Reboot Your Health: Simple DIY Tests and Solutions to Assess and Improve your Health' available on Amazon for a comprehensive strategy to identify and resolve any issues you may or may not be aware of, naturally and non-invasively.

Statistics: Statistics from Italy looking at 18% of the total COVID-19 deaths indicate that 99% of the people who died had underlying medical conditions. A quarter of those studied had one or two serious issues, and nearly a half of the victims had three or more health problems.

76.1% had high blood pressure
35.5% had diabetes
33% had heart problems.[19]

How to eat: Intermittent fasting is a method of controlling your food intake throughout the day, restricting your eating to a 6-8 hour window every 24 hours. It's easy to do: you can skip breakfast and simply eat two meals between 1pm and 7pm which will trigger a host of health benefits. Make sure, however, that you stop any food consumption at least three hours before you go to sleep.

Research shows that intermittent fasting improves blood sugar levels and boosts insulin sensitivity, which can help reduce high blood pressure and obesity and resolve Type 2 diabetes over time. It also reduces fatty liver.[20]

What to eat: For optimal energy levels, reduce the amount of carbohydrates you eat each day. Avoid sugars and instead eat fruits, vegetables, beans, lentils, lean proteins and healthy fats. Avoid eating snacks throughout the day, and not in the late evenings. Cut down on alcohol.

Balance your hormones

The second area to consider is that of hormonal imbalance. Severity of patients coronavirus symptoms has been linked to low levels of certain hormones. Dr Dario Acuna, Europe's leading expert on melatonin, is trialling high doses on COVID-19 patients and recommends increasing oral doses of melatonin both during infection and after. Melatonin is an immune system stimulator and reduces inflammation and oxidative stress.[21]

For the majority of patients, upping DHEA is vital. It is effective for reducing high blood pressure, insulin resistance and stress and anxiety levels. It boosts brain health and improves mood and sleep. It also strengthens immunity and increases the levels of T and NK cells and has been shown to improve the production of protective antibodies.[22]

Keeping cortisol levels in balance will help to regulate inflammation and keep anxiety levels down. Too much cortisol in the blood, released by feelings of stress and fear, can lower your immunity and overload your body's defensive systems. Try meditating daily to support your endocrine system, manage your hormone balance and sort your sleep. Deep breathing exercises will achieve a similar result. Download the Calm app, or see Wim Hof's breathing technique below.

Boost your immune system

The third key to a more rapid recovery is to boost your cell health in every way possible. Supplement, supplement and supplement some more, and keep taking vitamins and minerals in large quantities every day. The healthier your cells are, the less likely any virus will successfully re-invade them. (See Chapter Seven for anti-viral supplements).

Strategies to help to reboot your mitochondria, those tiny cellular ''energy batteries' that power your body are essential for getting back your energy. When you are physically and mentally exhausted, your body needs boosting with whatever you have to hand that might mop up residual viral infection and inflammation.

Wim Hof's breathing technique

Wim Hof is the world famous 'Ice Man' who developed a breathing technique that floods your body with oxygen, giving you the ability to alkalise your body and consciously control your immune system to fight off diseases. Just a few minutes every day gives you more energy, better sleep at night, reduced stress and a heightened immune response that helps to fight off viruses and recover from them faster. It's an inexpensive and effective way to re-invigorate your lungs and oxygenate the mitochondria.[23]

How to do it: Sit comfortably and breathe in deeply 30 to 40 times, inhaling through your nose and exhaling through your mouth. Then, take a deep breath and exhale; hold until you can't hold any longer and you need to breathe in. Inhale one more time, as deeply as you can, and hold again for 10 seconds before releasing. Do five sets in a row.

Drink hydrogen water

Hydrogen water is pure water with extra hydrogen molecules added to it. These molecular hydrogen molecules are so minute that they can cross the blood-brain barrier, accessing your cell membranes and protecting and reinvigorating your DNA and the mitochondria inside your cells. In a nutshell, this is super charged energy food for your mitochondria.

The science shows that hydrogen water is beneficial for overall immune system health, exactly what is needed during recovery. Research indicates that it is a powerful anti-oxidant. It improves your body's ability to absorb nutrients, it is anti-inflammatory,[24] it increases blood circulation and hydration levels and improves memory. And best of all in these post coronavirus days - indeed in all post viral infection recovery days - it does exactly what seems to be needed. It boosts energy.[25]

Passed as 'safe' by the USA FDA, you can make your own by investing in a hydrogen water machine, or simply add 2 hydrogen water tablets to your water bottle once a day.

Nebulising with hydrogen peroxide

> **Warning:** Hydrogen peroxide can be dangerous if misused. Please consult your doctor if you have health issues. Do not use any solution higher than 3%.

I have discussed the value of nebulizers on p78, but want to flag them again as a useful tool during your recovery period. Hydrogen peroxide is considered helpful for any lung weakness, a symptom experienced by many who have been affected by this virus.[26]

Airborne viruses of all types, whether a variant of the common cold, flu or the current COVID-19 pandemic, access your body via your mouth, nose or eyes. They hide in the mucous of your nasal passages, sinuses and airways, multiplying and as they do so triggering coughs, headaches, sore throats and blocked or runny noses. Then they move on deep into your lungs, causing breathing difficulties and ultimately sometimes pneumonia.

Nebulizers are mechanised pumps that you can use at home. They take a liquid, which can be a saline solution or a medicine, and turn it into a vapour mist that can be breathed in easily, reaching deep into your lungs. Rather like the Heineken ad, a nebulizer can reach the parts other sprays and potions simply cannot.

Hydrogen peroxide is a combination of hydrogen and water ($H2O2$). Chemically, it is simply water with another oxygen molecule added. It is antiseptic and kills bacteria, moulds and viruses. It oxygenates and detoxes your body.

Safe, easy to use and inexpensive, liquid hydrogen peroxide is effective for clearing and strengthening the mucous in your upper respiratory system and the lungs. Inhaling hydrogen peroxide as a fine vapour loosens the mucous build up in your lungs, lettings you cough it up and breathe more easily. No virus can survive in an oxygen rich environment, so getting additional oxygen to your lungs is key.

If you buy a bottle to use with your nebulizer, make sure you read the back carefully. It needs to be 3% food grade hydrogen peroxide and the ingredients listed should only be hydrogen peroxide and distilled water - no stabilisers of any kind. Don't take the 12% or 25% versions unless you are very good at maths and quantities and are able to accurately dilute down with distilled water to that 3%.

For some people, even 3% may feel too strong, so if you experience a slight burning sensation as you breathe then dilute down to 1.5% or even lower.

As a spray: If you can't, for whatever reason, get hold of a nebulizer, you can still put 3% hydrogen peroxide into an empty spray bottle (dilute it further with distilled water if it feels too strong at that %) and spray up your nose and to back of throat. It's not going to be as effective and penetrating as nebulizer but still an excellent protective solution and far better than doing nothing to protect your airways and clear your lungs.

Google 'Hydrogen Peroxide Inhalation Method by Bill Munro' who used it daily for decades to manage his lung conditions for further information on how and why it works. Or read up about it on my blog www.reboothealth.co.uk.

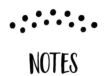

NOTES

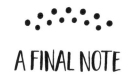

A FINAL NOTE

As research on COVID-19 continues to emerge over the months and years to come, we will get clearer answers as to how best to conquer this devastating infection. And if, as many scientist fear, we can't overcome it entirely and it mutates from year to year, then we will find out how to minimise the severity of our symptoms and optimise the speed of our recovery from it. Science will find a vaccine, and we will as a population develop anti-bodies that will boost our resistance. Together, we will get through it.

Right now that way forward is not clear, but in the meantime we can fall back on decades of research to use natural remedies to stay strong and build our immune systems.

I hope that the information in this book proves helpful to you and to your families and friends.

Stay safe, stay well. With my very best wishes,

Sara x

Sara Davenport writes the healthblog www.reboothealth.co.uk.

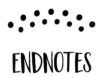

ENDNOTES

Introduction

1. E Yarnell 'Herbs for Emerging Viral Infectious Diseases' Alt and Complementary Therapies Aug 1 2016 164-174 Vol 22 Issue 4)

Chapter 1: All About Viruses

1. M Woolhouse 'Human viruses: discovery and emergence' Philos Trans R Soc Lond B Biol Sci 2012 Oct 19;367(1604):2864-2871

2. Sci/Tech planet bacteria – BBC news Tuesday Aug 25 1998)

3. Countryman J et al 'Stimulus duration and response time independently influence the kinetics of lytic cycle re-activation of Epstein-Barr virus'. J Virol 2009;83(20):10694-709

Chapter 2: Action Plan: How to Avoid a Virus

1. Kwok YL 'Face touching: a frequent habit that has implications for hand hygiene' Am J Infect Control 2015 Feb;43(2):112-4

2. N van Doremalen et al 'Aerosol and Surface Stability of SARS-CoV-2 as compared with SARS-CoV-1' New England Journal of Medicine March 17, 2020

3. Cunrui Huang et al 'The Hygienic Efficacy of Different Hand-drying methods: a review of the evidence' Mayo Clinic Proceedings August 2012 Volume 87, Issue 8, p 791-798.

4. 'Manchester biotech firm announces 'germ-trap' snood' 23 March 2020. businesscloud.co.uk

5. 'Cold plasma inactivates 99.9% of airborne viruses' 15 April 2019 Cleanroom technology

Chapter 3: Your In-Built Anti-Viral Protection

1. D Baxter 'Active and passive immunity, vaccine types, excipients and licensing' Occupational Medicine, Vol 57, Issue 8, Dec 2007, p552-556

2. T Kim et al 'Vaccine herd effect' Scand J Infect Dis. 2011 Sep; 43(9): 683–689

Chapter 4: Immune System Action Plan

1. B Azevedo 'Toxic effects of Mercury on the cardiovascular and central nervous systems' J Biomed Biotechnol 2012 July 2

2. Professor Chris Exley 'Why everyone should drink silicon-rich mineral water' Mental Health, Neurology, Nursing 15th March 2017

3. Qin et al 2010

4. Imad al Kassaa 'New Insights on antiviral Probiotics' Dec 2016 Springer ISBN-13 9783319496870

5. H Goto et al – Anti-influenza virus effects of both live and non-live Lactocillus acidophilu L-92 accompanied by the activation of innate immunity' British Journal of Nutrition 110(10), 1810-1818

6. T Kawashima 'Lactobacillus plantarum strain YU from fermented foods activates Th1 and protective immune responses' Int Immunopharmacology Vol 11 Issue 12 Dec 2011, p2017-2024

7. S Gabryszewski et al 'Lactobacillus-mediated priming of the respiratory mucosa protects against lethal pneumovirus infection' J Immunol, 186(2);1151-61

8. M Segers et al 'Towards a better understanding of Lactobacillus rhamnosus GG -host interactions' Microb Cell Fact 2014;13:S7

9. S Gabryszewski et al 'Lactobacillus-mediated priming of the respiratory mucosa protects against lethal pneumovirus infection' J Immunol, 186(2);1151-61

10. H Youn 'Intranasal administration of live lactobacillus species facilitates proection against influenza virus infection in mice' Antiviral Research, Vol 93 Issue 1, Jan 2012 p138-43

11. N West 'Lactobacillus fermentum supplementation and gastrointestinal and respiratory-tract illness symptoms: a randomised control trial in althletes. Nutrition Journal 10, Article 30 (2011)

12. K Shida et al 'Daily Intake of Fermented Milk with L Casei strain Shirota reduces the incidence and duration of Upper Respiratory Tract infections in Healthy Middle Aged Office workers' Eur J nutr Feb 2017

13. S Ooi et al 'Evidence-based Review of BioBran/MGN-3 Arabinoxylan Compound as a Complementary Therapy for conventional cancer Treatment' Integr Cancer Ther 2018 June;17(2):165-178

14. Khalid A et al 'Bactericidal and antibiotic synergistic effect of nanosilver against methicillin-resistant Staphylococcus aureus' Jundishapur Journal of Microbiology 2015 Nov;8(11):e25867

15. The Antimicrobial Activity of Selected Silver Products' R Rowen et al.

16. G Hollander et al 'Emerging Strategies to boost thymic function' Curr Opin Pharmacol 2010 Aug;10(4):443-453

17. A Lardner 'The effects of extracellular pH on immune function' J Leukoc Biol 2001 Apr;69(4):522-30

18. L Liang-Tzung et al 'Anti-viral Natural Products and Herbal Medicines' J Tradit Complement Med 2014 Jan-Mar;4(1):24-35

19. Armstrong ML et al 'Potassium initiates vasodilatation induced by a single skeletal muscle contraction in hamster cremaster muscle.' J Physiol. 2007 Jun 1;581(Pt 2):841-52

20. Chian LC et al 'Antiviral activities of extracts and selected pure constituents of Ocimum basilicum' Clin Exp Pharmacol Physiol 2005;32:811-6

21. S Rennard et al 'Chicken Soup Inhibits Neutrophil Chemotaxis in Vitro' Chest 2000 118:1150-1157

22. Ali A et al 'Curcumin inhibits HIV-1 by promoting Tat protein degradation.' Sci Rep 6:27539 2016

23. Maher D et al 'Curcumin suppresses human papilloma virus oncoproteins..'Mol Carcinog 50. 47-57

24. Chen T et al 'Inhibition of enveloped viruses infectivity by curcumin' PLOS One 8

25. Rehin et al 2016 'Curcumin and Boswellia Serrata gum resin extract inhibit chikungunya and vesicular stomatitis virus infections in vitro' Antiviral Res 125 51-57

26. D Praditya 'Anti-infective Properties of the Golden Spice Curcurmin' Frontiers in Microbiology 2019;10:912

27. JS Chang ' Fresh ginger has anti-viral activity against human respiratory syncytial virus in human respiratory tract cell lines' J Ethnopharmacol 2013 Jan 9;145(1):146-51

28. Garcia Larsen V et al 'Dietary antioxidants and 10-year lung function decline in adults from the ECRHS survey'. Eur Respir J. 2017 Dec 21;50(6)

29. 'A diet High in Saturated Fat and Cholesterol Accelerates Simian Immunodeficiency Virus Disease Progression' J infect Dis 2007 Oct 15:196(8):1202-10

Chapter 5: Sleep Action Plan

1. H Linn et al 'Effect of kiwifruit consumption on sleep quality in adults with sleep problems'. Asia Pac J Clin Nutr. 2011;20(2)

Chapter 6: Exercise Action Plan

1. A Coghland 'Best anti-ageing exercise is high intensity interval training' New Scientist 7 March 2017.

2. K Stokes et al 'The time course of the human growth hormone response to a 6 s and a 30 s cycle ergometer sprint' Journal of Sports Sciences 20(6):487-94· June 2002

3. Hartig, T et al 'Tracking restoration in natural and urban field settings'. Journal of Environmental Psychology, 2003 23(2), 109–123

Chapter 7: Anti-viral Nutritional Supplements

1. Te Velthuis et al, PLoS Pathog. 2010 Nov 4;6(11):e1001176. doi: 10.1371/journal.ppat.1001176. 'Zn(2+) inhibits coronavirus and arterivirus RNA polymerase activity in vitro and zinc ionophores block the replication of these viruses in cell culture'.

2. 'Impact of Trace Elements and Vitamin Supplementation on Immunity and Infections in Institutionalized Elderly PatientsA Randomized Controlled Trial' Francois Girodon et al Arch Intern Med. April 12 1999;159(7):748-754.

3. 'Zinc lozenges and the common cold: a meta-analysis comparing zinc acetate and zinc gluconate, and the role of zinc dosage' Harri Hemilä JRSM May 2 2017

4. 'Vitamin C Infusion for the Treatment of Severe 2019-nCoV Infected Pneumonia' Zhi Yong Peng, Zhongnan Hospital US National Library of Medicine Clinical trials.gov

5 Levy TE. 'Curing the incurable: Vitamin C, infectious diseases and toxins. 2011. Amazon.

6. 'N-acetyl cysteine functions as a fast-acting antioxidant by triggering intracellular H2S and sulfane sulfur production' D Ezerina et al Cell Chem Biiol 2018 April 19:25(4):447-459

7. Shing-Hwa Huang et al 'Melatonin possesses an anti-influenza potential through its immune modulatory effect' Journal of Functional Foods Vol 58, July 2019 p 189-198)

8. Hashemipour M et al 'Antiviral Activities of Honey, Royal Jelly and Acyclovir against HSV-1' Wounds 2014 Feb;26(2):47-54

9. Journal of Alternative and Complementary medicine – 'Intravenous Micronutrient therapies (Myers cocktail) for Fibromyalgia: a placebo-controlled pilot study Ather Ali et Al

Chapter 8: Harness the Power of Plants

1. P Schnitzler 'Antiviral activity of Australian tea tree oil and eucalyptus oil against herpes simplex virus in cell culture'. Pharmazie. 2001 Apr;56(4):343-7.

2. D Gilling et al 'Antiviral efficacy and mechanisms of action of oregano essential oil and its primary component carvacrol against murine norovirus'. J Appl Microbiol. 2014 May;116(5):1149-63

3. A Brochot 'Antibacterial, antifungal and antiviral effects of three essential oil blends' Microbiologyopen 2017 Aug; 6(4)e00459

4. A Brochot 'Antibacterial, antifungal and antiviral effects of three essential oil blends' Microbiologyopen 2017 Aug; 6(4)e00459

5. M K Swarmy et al.' Antimicrobial Properties of Plant Essential Oils against Human Pathogens and Their Mode of Action: An Updated Review' Evid Based Complement Alternat Med. 2016; 2016.

6. A Astani et al 'Screening for antiviral activities of isolated compounds from essential oils'. Evid Based Complement Alternat Med. 2011;2011:253643.

7. C Adams 'Thyme Antiviral Against Herpes and Other Viruses' Journal of plant medicines. Oct 3 2017

8. Hwa-Jung Choi 'Chemical Constituents of Essential Oils Possessing Anti-Influenza A/WS/33 Virus Activity' Osong Public Health Res Perspect. 2018 Dec; 9(6): 348–353

9. Amandine Brochot et al Antibacterial, antifungal, and antiviral effects of three essential oil blends Evid Based Complement Alternat Med. 2016; Published online 2016 Dec 20.
Mallappa Kumara Swamy, Antimicrobial Properties of Plant Essential Oils against Human Pathogens and Their Mode of Action: An Updated Review Microbiologyopen. 2017 Aug; 6(4): e00459.

Kampf G, Kramer A. Epidemiologic background of hand hygiene and evaluation of the most important agents for scrubs and rubs. Clin Microbiol Rev. 2004 Oct;17(4):863-93.

Yang Y., He H., Chang H., Yu Y., Yang M., He Y. Multivalent oleanolic acid human serum albumin conjugate as nonglycosylated neomucin for influenza virus capture and entry inhibition. Eur. J. Med. Chem. 2018;143:1723–1731.

10. Yuxi Liang et al ' Astragalus Membranaceus Treatment Protects Raw264.7 cells from Influenza virus by regulating G1 Phase and the TLR3-Mediated Signalling Pathway' Article ID 2971604 Dec 2019 Evidence Based complementary and Alternative Medicine

11. Aquino R et al 'Plant metabolites: New compounds and anti-inflammatory activity of Uncaria tomentosa (Cats Claw' J Nat Prod 1991;54(2):453-459)

(Aquino R et al ' 'Structure and in vitro antiviral activity of quinovic acid glycosides from Uncaria tomentosa and Guettarda platypoda' J Nat Prod 1989;52(4):679-685

12. Z Zakay-Rones 'Randomised study of the efficacy and safety of oral elderberry extract in the treatment of Influenza A and B virus infections' J Int Med Res March-Apr 2004

13. D H Gilling et al 'Antiviral Efficacy and Mechanisms of action of oregano essential oil and its primary component carvacrol against murine Norovirus J Appl Microbiol May 2014 116(51149-63

14. Fabian M. Dayrit, Ph.D 'The Potential of Coconut Oil and its Derivatives as Effective and Safe Antiviral Agents Against the Novel Coronavirus (nCoV-2019)' Posted on January 31, 2020 Integrated Chemists of the Philippines

15. Bing Du Xue Bao 'Anti-virus research of triterpenoids in licorice' 2013 Nov:29(6):673-9 Chinese Journal of Virology

Eric Yarnell 'Herbs for emerging viral infectious diseases' 1 Aug 2016 Alternative and Complementary Therapies Vol 22, No 4

16. Johanna Signer et al 'In vitro antiviral activity of Echinaforce, an Echinacea purpurea preparation, against common cold coronavirus 229E and highly pathogenic MERS-CoV and SARAS-CoV' Virology Journal 26 Feb 2020

17. 'Broad-spectrum anti-viral properties of andrographolide' Archives of Virology. Vol 162 p 611-625

18. 'Oleuropein in Olive and its Pharmacological Effects' Syed Haris Omar, College of Pharmacy, Qassim University 23 April 2010

19. P Samuel et al 'Stevia Leaf to Stevia Sweetner: Exploring its science, benefits and future potential' Journal of Nutrition Vol 148, Issue 7, July 2018 P 1186S-1205S

20. S A Kedikk et al 'Antiviral activity of dried extract of Stevia' Pharmaceutical Chemistry Journal 43(4):198-199 April 2009.

21. A Vela 'Anti HIV activity of extracts from Calendula officinalis leaves infected by an anisometric virus' Microbiol Esp Jan-Mar 1970 23(1);47-60

22. MD Mandal 'Honey: its medicinal property and antibacterial activity, Asian Pacific Journal of Tropical Biomedicine 154 2011;1(2):154-160.

Chapter 9: Air, Ozone And Heat

1. D Posa et al . 'Efficacy and usability of a novel nebulizer targeting both upper and lower airways' Italian Journal of Pediatrics 29 September 2017

2. M A Baugh 'HIV: reactive oxygen species, enveloped viruses and hyperbaric oxygen' Med hypotheses 2000 Sept;55(3):232-8

3. Kohen R et al 'Oxidation of biological systems:oxidative stress phenomena, antioxidantsm, redox reactions, and methods for their quantification' Toxicol Pathol 2002 Nov-Dec;30(6):620-50

4. A M Elvis et al 'Ozone therapy: A clinical review' J Nat Sci Biol Med 2011 Jan-Jun;2(1);66-70
   J B Hudson 'Development of a Practical Method for Using Ozone Gas as a Virus Decontaminating Agent' Ozone:Science & Engineering, Vol 31, 2009 – Issue 4 27 May 2009 p216-223

5. N van Doremalen et al 'Stability of Middle East respiratory syndrome coronavirus (MERS-CoV) under different environmental conditions' Eurosurveillance Vol 18 Issue 38 19/Sept/2013

6. WHO Coronavirus disease 2019 (COVID-19) Situation Report – 32 21 February 2020

7. J Hussain 'Clinical Effects of Regular Dry Sauna Bathing: a systemic review' Hindawi Volume 2018 Article ID 1857413 24 April 2018

8. J Johnson 'What are the benefits of a steam room?' Medical News Today Dec 15 2017

9. J Hudson 'Echinacea – 'A source of potent antivirals for respiratory virus infections' Pharmaceuticals 2011 Jul:4(7):1019-1031

10. V Micol 'The olive leaf extract exhibits antiviral activity against viral haemorrhagic septicaemia rhabdovirus (VHSV)'. Antiviral Res. 2005 Jun;66(2-3):129-36. Epub 2005 Apr 18.

11. Erowele GI, Kalejaiye AO. 'Pharmacology and therapeutic uses of cat's claw'. American Journal of Health-System Pharmacy. 2009;66(11):992-995.

12. L Macedo et al 'ß-Lapachone activity in synergy with conventional antimicrobials against methicillin resistant Staphylococcus aureus strains'. Phytomedicine. 2013 Dec 15;21(1):25-9.

Chapter 10: Action Plan: Anti-viral Home Solutions

1. J Greatorex et al 'Effectiveness of common household cleaning agents in reducing the viability of Human Influenza A/H1N1' Plos One Feb 1 2010

2. N van Doremalen, et al. 'Aerosol and surface stability of HCoV-19 (SARS-CoV-2) compared to SARS-CoV-1.'The New England Journal of Medicine. DOI: 10.1056/NEJMc2004973 (2020)

3. L Dimugno 'Disinfectants: A guide to killing germs the right way' MNN.com/Health/Healthy spaces. March 6 2020

4. J Greatorex et al 'Effectiveness of Common Household Cleaning Agents in Reducing the Viability of Human Influenza A/H1N1' PlosOne Feb 1 2010

5. Edmonds-Wilson SL 'Review of human hand microbiome research' J Dermat Sci 2015 Oct;80(1):3-12

6. Lukasik J, et al 'Reduction of poliovirus 1, bacteriophages, Salmonella montevideo, and Escherichia coli O157:H7 on strawberries by physical and disinfectant washes.'J Food Prot. 2003 Feb;66(2):188-93

Chapter 11: Emotions and Immunity

1. Music as medicine? 30 minutes a day shows benefits after heart attack' American college of cardiology March 18 2020
2. N Leigh Hunt et al 'An overview of systematic reviews on the public health consequences of social isolation and loneliness' Public Health Vol 152 Nov 2017 p157-171

Chapter 12: Stress Relief: Unload Your Burden

1. Holmes Rahe stress inventory Occupational Medicine 2017;67:581–582 doi:10.1093/occmed/kqx099
2. Léia Fortes Salles et al 'Effect of flower essences in anxious individuals' Acta paul. enferm. vol.25 no.2 São Paulo 2012
3. Hoge EA 'Randomized controlled trial of mindfulness meditation for generalized anxiety disorder: effects on anxiety and stress reactivity' J Clin Psychiatry. 2013 Aug;74(8):786-92. doi: 10.4088/JCP.12m08083.
4. Amy Serin et al 'The therapeutic Effect of Bilateral Alternating Stimulation Tactile Form Technology on the Stress Response' Journal of Biotechnology and Biomedical Science. Issn No:2576-6694
5. C Sweeney 'A traditional therapy finds modern uses' New York Times Feb 21 2008 www.simplyacupuncture.co.uk

Chapter 13: Coronavirus – a global pandemic

1. Vital Surveillances: The epidemiological characteristics of an Outbreak of 2019 Novel Coronavirus Diseases (COVID-19)' Feb 18 2020 Chinese Center for Disease Control and Prevention
2. S Lauer et al ' The Incubation Period of Coronavirus Disease 2019 (COVID-19) from Publicly Reported Confirmed Cases: Estimation and Application' Ann Intern Med 2020 10 March
3. J Oke et al 'Global Covid-19 Case Fatality Rates' CEBM 21 March 2020
4. Vanessa Bates Ramirez 'What is R0? Gauging Contagious Infections' University of Illinois-Chicago, College of Medicine June 24, 2016
5. WHO Q&A on coronaviruses (COVID-19) 'Can I catch COVID-19 from my pet? 9 March 2020
6. 'W Guan et al 'Clinical Characteristics of Corona Disease 2019 in China' New England Journal of Medicine Feb 28 2020
7. Report of the WHO-China Joint Mission on Coronavirus Disease 2019 (COVID-19)
8. E Keyaets et al 'Antiviral Activity of Chloroquine against Human Coronavirus OC43 Infection in new born mice' Antimicrobial Agents and Chemotherapy DOI:10.1128/AAC.01509-08
Savarino A et al 'Effects of chloroquine on viral infections: an old drug against todays diseases?' Lancet Infect Dis 3:722-727

9. Favirpiravir. Justin mcCurry 'Japanese flu drug 'clearly effective' in treating coronavirus, says China'. The Guardian. 18 March 2020

10. Remdisivir. Abby Olena 'Remdesivir Works Against Coronaviruses in the Lab' 'The antiviral disables RNA replication machinery in MERS and SARS viruses. Can it beat back SARS-CoV-2?' The Scientist. Mar 20, 2020

11. M Day 'Covid 19: 'Ibuprofen should not be used for managing symptoms say doctors and scientists BMJ 2020; 368 17 March 2020

12. M Bhatia 'Coronavirus Covid-19 – 'Analysis of symptoms from confirmed cases with an assessment of possible homeopathic remedies for treatment and prophylaxis' March 4 20202 Know Your Disease

13. R Woelfel 'Clinical presentation and virological assessment of hospitalized cases of coronavirus disease 2019 in a travel-associated transmission cluster' oi: https://doi.org/10.1101/2020.03.05.20030502

14. H Hakimullah et al 'Evaluation of sprayed hypochlorous acid solutions for their virucidal activity against avian influenza virus through in vitro experiments' J Vet Med Sci. 2015 Feb; 77(2): 211–215

15. John Scott Meschke Professor and Director of Environmental and Occupational Health Microbiology Lab Department of Environmental and Occupational Health Sciences School of Public Health, University of Washington. 3/4/2016). Also Rasmussen, E 'Stabilised hypochlorous acid disinfection for highly vulnerable populations: Brio HOCL wound disinfection and area decontamination' 2017 IEEE Global Humanitarian Technology conference.)

16. Thermographic Evaluation of the MRET-Shield Polymer on the Reduction of Thermal Effects Caused by Radio Frequency Radiation' Explore Magazine, Vol.18, No.1: 14-17

17. Ref Weinberg, E et al ' Humming greatly increases nasal nitric oxide'. American Journal of respiratory and critical care medicine 166.2 2002:144-45

18. Jamison J et al 'Critical role for the NLRP3 inflammasome during acute lung injury'. J Immunol 2014 June 15; 192(12):5974-5983

19. Istituto Superiore di Sanita 'Characteris+cs of COVID-19 pa+ents dying in Italy' 17 April 2020

20. De Cabo et al 'Effects of intermittent fasting on health, ageing and disease' New England Journal of Medicine, Dec 2019.

21. Boga, JA et al 'Beneficial actions of melatonin in the management of viral infections: a new use for this 'molecular handyman'. Rev Med Virol 2012 Sept;22(5):323-38.

22. Prall, S et al 'DHEA modulates immune function: A review of evidence' Vitamins and Hormones 2018 125-144.

23. M Kox et al 'Voluntary activation of the sympathetic nervous system and attenuation of the innate immune response in humans' Proc Natl Acad Sci USA May 20 2014

24. Guohua Song et al 'Hydrogen-rich water decreases serum LDL-cholesterol levels and improves HDL function in patients with potential metabolic syndrome' J Lipid Res. 2013 Jul; 54(7): 1884–1893.

25. 'Open-label trial and randomized, double-blind, placebocontrolled, crossover trial of hydrogen-enriched water for mitochondrial and inflammatory myopathies'.Med Gas Res. 2011 Oct 3;1(1):24.

26. American Thoracic Society 'Inhaling hydrogen may help reduce lung damage in critically ill patients, animal study suggests' May 16 2011.

INDEX

A

Acupressure 117, 127
AcuPips 117
Air 76-82, Air Filtration 13
Alcohol 44, 50
Alkalising 38
Allitech 43
Aloe vera gel 88
Animals 30, 122
Antibiotics 17
Antibodies 17
Anti-viral drugs 17
Apples 43
Apple cider vinegar 129
Astragalus 70

B

Bach Flower Remedies 111
Bacteria 4
Baking soda 87, 91
Bananas 39
Baseline Testing 24
Bicarbonate of Soda 87, 91
Biobran 34
Blood pressure high 24
Bone marrow 19

C

Calendula 75
Cardiovascular disease 24
Castor oil 50
Cats Claw 71, 85
Chemicals 28
Chicken soup 41-42
Chronic respiratory illness 24
Cinnamon 68, 69, 87
Circadian rhythms 51
Cleaning 10, 11
    mobile phones 12
    fruit & veg 12
    petrol station 15
    surfaces 86
Cloroquine 125
Close contact 11, 12
Clove 68, 69
Coconut oil 72
Colloidal silver 36-37
COPD 79

Coronavirus 119-138
Cortisol 135
Coughing 10
Curcumin 42, 65

D

Dairy 43
DHEA 134
Diabetes 24
Diet 39-44
Diffuser 82
DMSO 65
Doctors 15
Dr Munshi breathing 116

E

Echinacea 73
EFT 107, 131
Elderberry 71
Essential Oils 66-70
Eucalyptus 67, 87
Exercise 52-57

F

Fats 43
Favipirivir 125
Fermented foods 40
Fever 20

G

Gargling 83
Garlic 42
Ginger 42
Green tea 85

H

Hair Mineral Analysis Test 26
Handwashing 10
Headache 131
Herd immunity 21
High Intensity Interval Training (HIIT) 54-55
HOCL 130
Homeopathy 126-127
Hormones 134
Humming 130
Hydrogen peroxide 64, 137-139

Hydrogen water 136

I

Immune system 17-44
Immunity 20
Inhalation 83
Intermittent fasting 134
Intravenous therapy 63-65
Isolation 97

J

Juices 40

K

Kiwi fruit 50

L

Liquorice root 72
Lymphatic system 19

M

Magnesium 49
Manuka Honey 75
Masks 14
Meditation 94, 113-115, 134
Mental Health Apps 108
Melatonin 62, 134
Mould 26-27
Myers cocktail 64

N

NAC 61
Nebulizer 78, 136
New habits 9-13

O

Ogden Home Health Kit 23
Olive Leaf 74, 85
On Guard Oil 69
Oregano 67, 72
Oxidation 80
Oxygen 77-78
    oxygen meter 77
    Hyperbaric 79
    Vital Air therapy 79
Ozone 79-80

P

Panic 15
Paracetamol 126
Parasites 29-30
Pau D'Arco 85
Pets 30, 119
Probiotics 30-34
Proning 128
Propolis 129, 130
Pulse oximeter 132

R

Ravensara Aromatica 70
Ravintsara 70
Remdesivir 125
R0 number 120
Rosemary 68, 69, 87
Royal Jelly 62

S

Sauna 83
Sage 68
Self-isolation 124
Silver Hydrosol 65, 67
Sleep 45-51
Social distancing 124
Sodium Bicarbonate 65
Sore throat 83, 128
SOS Advance 69
Spleen 19
Star Anise 68
Steam 84
Stevia 74
Stress 7, 100-116
Supplements 62
Sweet Basil 40

T

Tapping 107
Teas 84-85
Tea tree oil 88, 128
Temperature 9, 82
Thieves Oil 69
Thyme 68
Thymus 18,19, 37-38
Touchpoints 117
Toxic metals 25, 26

V

Vaccines 17, 20
Valerian 49
Vitamins
    A 60
    B 65
    C 61,65
    D 58-59
    K 59
Vitamin E oil 88
Virus 3-8, 71
    Coronavirus 116-127
Viral load 8
    The problem with 20

W

Water, Acilis 26
Washing clothes 92
Wheatgrass 35
White blood cells 7, 17, 19, 34, 59, 64
WiFi 130
Wim Hof breathing 136
Working from home 98-99

Y

Yoga Nidra 116

Z

Zinc 59
Zinc lozenges 129

If you have enjoyed *Viral Self Defence*, why not add Sara Davenport's
Reboot Your Health and *Reboot Your Brain* to your library
of health favourites?

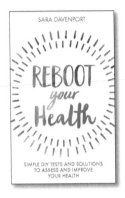 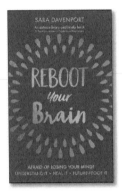

And if you would like to read in-depth articles on many of the
topics in these books, please sign up for the fortnightly newsletter
on www.reboothealth.co.uk and receive a free e-copy of my book
Understanding Alzheimer's which retails at £6.99.

Reboot Your Health looks at all aspects of holistic health and healing,
bringing you a regular dose of DIY get-well advice. From nutrition
to detox, sleep to air pollution and the best health tests on the
market, the blog covers a wide range of topics, delivering you the low-
down on conventional medicine and complementary therapies. Check
out the range of top tips, recipes and ideas on how to live better; sign
up today for information on a whole host of brain relevant topics and
find out about health experts who might just change your life. All free
of charge and backed by science.

All your questions answered on topics such as:

Air pollution, Brain Fog, Pesticides, Lyme disease, Sleep, Mould, Detox,
Candida, Electromagnetic fields and the arrival of 5G, Trigeminal
Neuralgia, Brain biotics, Dementia, Toxic teeth, HIIT and exercise,
Stem cells, Mental health apps

And many, many more.

Reboot Your Health – if you don't take care of yourself, who else is going to?

Printed in Great Britain
by Amazon